T0213534

Food and Health

Series Editors
Jonathan Deutsch, Drexel University, Philadelphia, PA, USA
Brandy-Joe Milliron, Drexel University, Philadelphia, PA, USA

The goal of this series is to provide coverage of emerging topics in food and health, using an interdisciplinary approach that considers health not only in a functional and human sense, but also in terms of external factors such as the environment. Titles in the series will address growing concerns about the future health, sustainability and quality of the food supply, as well as diet, and provide a home for books focusing on social and environmental concerns related to food.

More information about this series at https://springer.com/series/15394

Jeffrey P. Miller • Charlene Van Buiten

Editors

Superfoods

Cultural and Scientific Perspectives

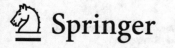 Springer

Editors
Jeffrey P. Miller
Department of Food Science & Human
Nutrition
Colorado State University
Fort Collins, CO, USA

Charlene Van Buiten
Colorado State University
Fort Collins, CO, USA

ISSN 2509-6389   ISSN 2509-6397   (electronic)
Food and Health
ISBN 978-3-030-93242-8   ISBN 978-3-030-93240-4   (eBook)
https://doi.org/10.1007/978-3-030-93240-4

This Springer imprint is published by the registered company Springer Nature Switzerland AG
The registered company address is: Gewerbestrasse 11, 6330 Cham, Switzerland

Preface – Superfoods

Superfoods are a topic of keen interest today. A Google search of the term will return over 70 million results in seconds. But what are superfoods? What qualities make a food a superfood? There is no regulated definition for the term in the United States, and the European Union (EU) specifically bans the use of the term in the marketing and promotion of food unless the EU has authorized a specific health claim for the food. The Oxford English Dictionary defines a superfood as "a nutrient-rich food considered to be especially beneficial for health and well-being." In the popular imagination, a superfood is one that has extremely high levels of a desired nutrient and/or a preventive or therapeutic health effect and has no negative consequences to its consumption.

Marketers are quick to seize on any study that purports a health benefit or special nutritive density to market a specific food as a superfood. Products that are perceived as healthier or "natural", another term with little or no regulation about its use, tend to bring higher prices in the marketplace.

Superfoods are often touted as a path to looking and feeling younger and having a healthier self. The Western diet and its overabundance of fat, salt, and sugar have increased the incidence of diet-related disease in the modern era. The idea that what we eat can lead to ill-health has created a great deal of nutritional anxiety in the Western consumer. Superfoods are often promoted as the remedy to this nutritional anxiety. This promotion is aided by the fact many people consider nutritional health to be a commodity that can be purchased at a monetary price, independent of the correlative factors contributed by other inputs. The notion exists that if one buys and eats a superfood, they will become a picture of glowing health.

Superfoods are not consumed solely for their nutritive value. Superfoods fit into a larger schema of health, self-image, and consumption popular with people in the upper-income tranches of highly developed nations. Superfoods are seen as "natural" alternatives to highly processed and fortified foods. The lore of production and consumption by exotic indigenous people in far-away lands who are superb stewards of the environment fulfills a social and ethical need for consumers in highly developed countries who consume the lion's share of the world's resources.

While superfoods may be ill-regulated and unable to live up to the hyperbole associated with them, they can be useful in modern diets when paired with under-standing of the specificities, nuances, and limitations of their benefits towards human health. The fact that many of them are eaten in lightly or unprocessed forms often make them better eating choices than the plethora of highly processed and fortified food choices available to the modern consumer. Conversely, the processing that must take place to create some superfoods such as tea, chocolate, and wine can enhance their benefits to the modern consumer. Superfoods as a category are an outgrowth of research on functional foods [foods with specific beneficial functions in the body], and there may well be good reason to consume foods with high levels of anti-oxidants, phytochemicals, and the like.

Contents

Chapter 1
Introduction to Superfoods

Jeffrey P. Miller

Superfoods. The term conjures up visions of vitality and longevity gained by the consumption of single potent foodstuff. While the idea of something being a super-food has gotten its greatest traction in the twenty-first century, the term has been around for at least a hundred years. According to the Harvard School of Public Health, the term superfood was first used in conjunction with a marketing campaign by the United Fruit Company (the corporate forerunner of Chiquita Brands International) to get people to eat more bananas (Harvard, 2021). Bananas were not only cheap, filling, nutritious, and culinarily appealing; they were also touted as cures for celiac disease and diabetes.

In a sense, the idea of superfood has always been with us. How superfoods are conceived and defined changes with a society's needs at places and times in history. The definition of the term is therefore somewhat malleable. The quest to find super-foods is probably closely tied to the human fascination with immortality. Humans live in two worlds, the symbolic and the natural. In the symbolic world, immortality is a potent concept and one that is widely attractive across cultures and beliefs. In the natural world there is little to suggest that immortality is attainable. The idea that a single foodstuff can improve vitality and extend longevity becomes a potent tool in the arsenal of those who wish to bridge the divide between the symbolic world and the natural world. Hence the fascination with something we have labelled a superfood.

Humans use many tools to deny and defy mortality. Some are tools of the mind – like art and philosophy and religion. Some are tools of the body – like medicine and nutrition and exercise. Humans appear to have been fascinated with the idea of

J. P. Miller (✉)
Colorado State University, Fort Collins, CO, USA
e-mail: Jeffrey.miller@colostate.edu

© The Author(s), under exclusive license to Springer Nature Switzerland AG 2022
J. P. Miller, C. Van Buiten (eds.), *Superfoods*, Food and Health,
https://doi.org/10.1007/978-3-030-93240-4_1

perfect health and immortality from very early times. Many folk tales and legends are concerned with health, longevity, and even immortality.

In the Garden of Eden, Adam and Eve are presented with two primary plants, the Tree of Life and the Tree of Knowledge. Consuming the fruit of the Tree of Life promised immortality while consuming the fruit of the Tree of Knowledge promised death (Haleem, 1997). Other early religions proffer similar ideas. In Greek mythology, consuming Ambrosia and Nectar provided immortality to the gods (Baratz, 2015). In Hindu ritual, drinking *Amrit* or *Soma* confers longevity or immortality and cures illness Ahamed et al., 2019). Examples of a certain food providing longevity, vitality, or even immortality exist in virtually every early culture.

Almost all early cultural tales about the possibility of becoming immortal connect the possibility with consuming some sort of foodstuff. Sometimes the foodstuff is hidden and likely unobtainable, as in the case of the plant of immortality found, then lost, by Gilgamesh (Nadolu & Nadolu, 2019). Other times longevity or immortality are contained in foods widely available such as the example of peaches in Chinese lore (Madihassan, 1984).

Any food that could confer immortality would surely be a superfood. While our generation has different ideas and immediate expectations for what would be called a superfood, the idea we have today is really not so different from the earliest ideas about the concept.

The original superfood is probably salt. Salt is needed for normal nerve and muscle function (Lewis, 2020). While societies in the pre-modern medicine era didn't understand the microbiology of salt in the body, they were capable observers of the effects of salt in the diet. People who got salt thrived and those who didn't get salt did not thrive.

Salt draws moisture from flesh and humans have long used salt as way to preserve precious animal flesh against times of need (Vandenriessche, 2008). Many of our favorite cultural food preferences like ham, bacon, and cured salmon have their beginnings in the need to preserve food for consumption outside of times of plenty. Jerky, lean meat that is salted and dehydrated, has an extremely long shelf, contra fresh meat which goes bad very quickly. These powers of preservation were practically magical in societies where a store of food that kept for long period time could mean the difference between starvation and survival. A steady source of salt was important enough to go to war for until fairly modern times. Salt production was so critical that many nations made it a government monopoly, with proceeds from salt sales funding many critical governmental expenditures (Cirrolo, 1994).

Another early superfood was sugar. Originating in New Guinea, sugar cane made its way to India where people learned to refine the juice from crushed cane into the crystalline form we are familiar with today (Abbott, 2010). Through the medieval period sugar was extremely expensive and in Europe it was valued more for its medicinal properties than its culinary possibilities. Writing in the twelfth century, William of Tyre described sugar as "'a most precious product, very necessary for the use and health of mankind' (Bronstein et al., 2019). The great sugar scholar Sid Mintz noted in "Sweetness and Power" that in this period, the English were using sugar as treatment for ailments as varied as chapped lips, fever, and several diseases of the chest and gut (Mintz, 1986).

Many alcoholic beverages that we enjoy today started out as sugar-sweetened medicines. In the days before germ theory and modern medical innovations, herbs were the primary components of most pharmecopia. Alcohol was used to make extracts and tinctures to concentrate the healing power of the herbs (Dubick, 1986). The resulting medicines were often extremely bitter and the pharmacists of the day frequently added sugar to make the medicine more palatable for the patient. Jagermeister Liqueur started out as a remedy for cough and digestion problems before entering the pantheon of popular social beverages. Sugar was a key element in many medicines in use before the nineteenth century. The practice was so widespread that the phrase "like an apothecary without sugar" came into use to describe an unthinkable or untenable situation (Fischler, 1987).

Throughout most of history, food and wellness have been strongly connected. While he may not have actually said it, we attribute the phrase *"let food be thy medicine and thy medicine be thy food"* to Hippocrates. The earliest version of the famous Hippocratic Oath we can find says *"I will use those dietary regimens which will benefit my patients according to my greatest ability and judgment, and I will do no harm or injustice to them"* (Hulkower, 2016).

From the third century CE until the seventeenth century, the most influential physician in the western world was Galen of Pergamon. Building on the works of Hippocrates and other Greek and Persian forbearers, Galen outlined a humoral system of medicine where illness was caused by an imbalance of the four humors – black bile, yellow bile, phlegm, and blood (Anderson, 1987). The way to return a body to the correct balance was through the consumption of food. Different foods had different properties, so if one had an overabundance of one humor, it would be corrected by eating a food from the opposing quadrant. In this system of medicine, any food could be a superfood if consuming it cured an ailment.

The invention of the compound microscope (two lenses) by the Jannsens, *per et fils,* could rightly be called the event that began the era of modern medicine (Hajdu, 2002). With the magnification made possible by these devices, early microscopists were able to see bacteria, protozoa, and epithelial cells. Improvements in these devices over the following two hundred years made possible the early discoveries by Pasteur, Fleming, and others that laid the basis for modern medicine.

While medical emphases shifted from nutrition to germ-theory in the nineteenth century, research on food and nutrition continued. Being able to see the smallest components of within our foods reoriented our food research focus from the macro to the micro. In the nineteenth century, food and nutrition research initially concentrated on fats, carbohydrates, and proteins, with some work in the area of minerals as well. Minerals like iodine, zinc, and iron were used to treat nutritional deficiencies with great success and could be considered an early example of a superfood (Mozaffarian, 2018).

In 1912 Casimir Funk coined the term *vitamins,* a portmanteau coinage of the terms *vital* and *amines.* Vitamin A was the first vitamin isolated in research, followed quickly by Vitamins B, C and D (Mozaffarian, 2018). Vitamin supplementation and fortification quickly became popular and vitamins are still thought of superfoods today, even though the emphasis has changed to whole food products containing them when using the term.

Research interest in micronutrients and phytochemicals began to grow with discoveries in the second half of the twentieth century. Micronutrients, as the name suggests, are substances that the body needs, but in very small amounts (Kotecha, 2008). Phytochemicals are chemicals that originate in plants and, though nonnutritive in and of themselves, provide health benefit to humans when consumed. While most human nutrition is provided by the macronutrients – lipids, proteins, and carbohydrates; micronutrients and phytochemicals provide beneficial health effects, though there may be risk in consuming large amounts of them through the use of concentrates and extracts (Craig, 1997). Nonetheless, many have been hailed as superfoods and plants that contain them are on many lists of superfoods today.

1.1 What We Eat

Living beings or organisms are usually classified into five kingdoms; animal, plant, fungi, protist, and monera (Verma, 2016). The human diet consists of foodstuffs from all of the five kingdoms of living things, plus a number of minerals. At one time or another, certain constituents of all of these kingdoms, and various minerals have been acclaimed as super foods. From the animal kingdom we mostly eat the lean muscle tissue and organs of various animals with endoskeletons, but we also consume animals with exoskeletons like shellfish and even animals without any skeleture such as jellyfish (Khong et al., 2016). In addition to muscle tissue and organs we consume animal collagens like we get from jellyfish and various fats and oils from these animals.

From the plant kingdom we eat a variety of plant parts, a practice sometimes dubbed "eating root to shoot" in a play on the "nose to tail" parlance popular with modern consumers. We commonly eat leaves, fruits, roots, and seeds of plants. With some plants we eat just one part, but many plants have multiple edible parts.

From the fungi kingdom we eat numerous mushrooms and edible fungi such as tree ears. Probably the most commonly consumed member of this kingdom is yeast. From the Protista family we eat seaweeds, which are multicellular Protista (Bajpai, 2019). Nori, the wrap used in sushi rolls and a component of other Japanese dishes is a Protista. From the Monera kingdom come edible blue-green algae. Spirulina, often touted as a superfood, is in the Monera kingdom (Kutala et al., 2008).

Minerals are important part of human nutrition and virtually all of them can be obtained through eating plants, animals, or members of the other three biological kingdoms. Living organisms obtain minerals from their environment and we consume them when we consume foodstuffs made from these organisms. Minerals can be obtained from sources that are not food products and minerals obtained this way are often used to fortify foods (Gutiontov, 2014). Examples of foods fortified with minerals include breakfast cereals and milk. Some of this fortification is required by law, but a good deal of it is discretionary.

1.2   How Are We Looking at So-Called Superfoods Today?

The term superfoods is not a medical or nutrition term in the strictest sense, but has become so widespread that it has been included in new editions of most of the dictionaries of the English Language. The Oxford English Dictionary defines a superfood as "a nutrient-rich food considered to be especially beneficial for health and well-being." In the popular imagination, a superfood is one that has extremely high levels of a desired nutrient and/or a chemopreventive or chemotherapeutic effect. Foods often get promoted to superfood status when a research report suggest that some component of the food is particularly effective in the prevention of disease, can affect significant weight loss, or improve mental health.

Today many consumers take Hippocrates advice to *"let food be thy medicine and thy medicine be thy food"* to heart. The foodservice consulting company Tastewise tells its customers that functional foods (sometimes referred to as nutraceuticals) are the fastest growing area of interest with food consumers. Health claims on food packages strongly influence consumer purchase decisions (UCDavis). Significant numbers of consumers with health problems such as diabetes, obesity, hypertension, and high cholesterol are actively attempting to manage their conditions through the use of functional foods.

The second decade of the twenty-first century saw a meteoric rise in the use of the term superfood in relation to prepared food and beverage products. "Old" superfoods like blueberries and green tea were joined by new names like acai, chia, and goji. Many of the foods that are touted as superfoods are indeed nutrient-dense at some level and likely can provide some health benefit when consumed. The problem with the designation is that many consumers will consume them disproportionately and neglect other vital areas of nutritional balance.

The interest in superfoods has never been higher, or so it seems. A Google search of the term in early 2021 returned over 220 million hits in less than 1 second. Information on superfoods on the internet covers the gamut, from the usually reliable like the Harvard Health Blog to hucksters claiming their superfood concoction will cure every condition from medical to sexual.

In the pages that follow we will look at a number of foods that are currently being touted as superfoods and examine them through historical and cultural lenses as well as scrutinizing the current state of nutritional research into them. Should you be interested in trying these foods for yourself, we will provide recipes using them for your consideration.

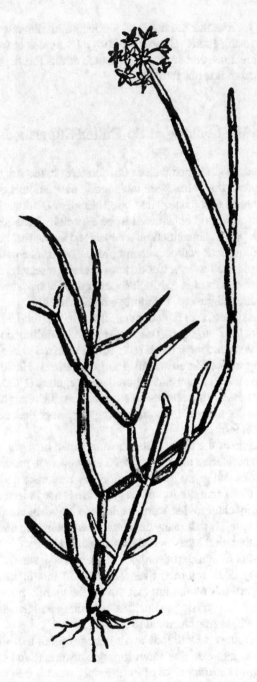

Soma Plant. (Romesh Chunder Dutt, Unknown author, Public domain, via Wikimedia Commons)

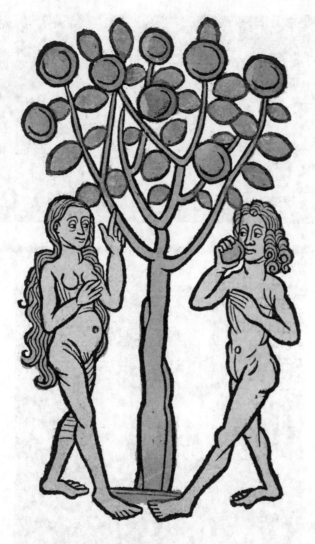

Tree of Life. (Unknown author, Public domain, via Wikimedia Commons)

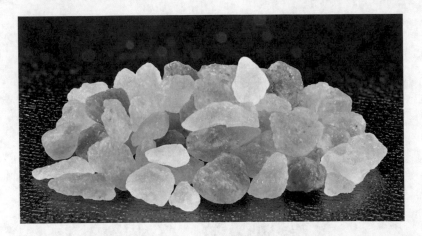

Salt Crystals. (Ivar Leidus, CC BY-SA 4.0 <https://creativecommons.org/licenses/by-sa/4.0>, via Wikimedia Commons)

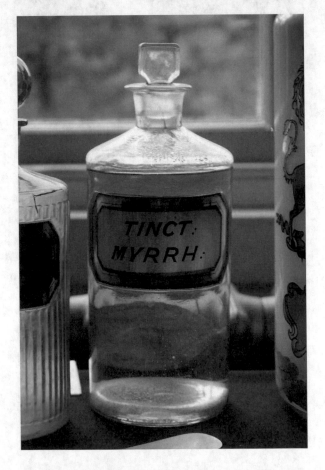

Tincture of Myrrh. (Stephencdickson, CC BY-SA 4.0 <https://creativecommons.org/licenses/by-sa/4.0>, via Wikimedia Commons)

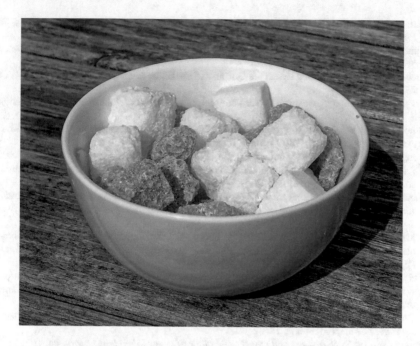

Sugar cubes. (Acabashi, CC BY-SA 4.0 <https://creativecommons.org/licenses/by-sa/4.0>, via Wikimedia Commons)

References

Abbott, E. (2010). *Sugar: A bittersweet history*. Bloomsbury Publishing.

Ahamed, S., Madan, P., & Singh, A. K. (2019). Transhumanism in India: Past, present and the future. In N. Lee (Ed.), *The transhumanism handbook*. Springer. https://doi.org/10.1007/978-3-030-16920-6_56

Anderson, E. N., Jr. (1987). Why is humoral medicine so popular? *Social Science & Medicine, 25*(4), 331–337.

Bajpai, P. (2019). Characteristics of algae. In *Third generation biofuels* (pp. 11–15). Springer.

Baratz, A. (2015). The source of the Gods' immortality in archaic Greek literature. *Scripta Classica Israelica, 34*, 151–164.

Bronstein, J., Stern, E. J., & Yehuda, E. (2019). Franks, locals and sugar cane: A case study of cultural interaction in the Latin Kingdom of Jerusalem. *Journal of Medieval History, 45*(3), 316–330.

Cirillo, M., Capasso, G., Di Leo, V. A., & De Santo, N. G. (1994). A history of salt. *American Journal of Nephrology, 14*(4–6), 426–431.

Craig, W. J. (1997). Phytochemicals: Guardians of our health. *Journal of the American Dietetic Association, 97*(10), S199–S204.

Dubick, M. A. (1986). Historical perspectives on the use of herbal preparations to promote health. *The Journal of Nutrition, 116*(7), 1348–1354.

Fischler, C. (1987). Attitudes towards sugar and sweetness in historical and social perspective. In *Sweetness* (pp. 83–98). Springer.

Gutiontov, S. (2014). Vital amines, purple smoke. A select history of vitamins and minerals. *The Pharos of Alpha Omega Alpha-Honor Medical Society, 77*, 18–24.

Hajdu, S. I. (2002). The first use of the microscope in medicine. *Annals of Clinical and Laboratory Science, 32*(3), 309–310.

Haleem, M. (1997). Adam and Eve in the Qur'an and the Bible. *Islamic Quarterly, London, 41*(4), 255. Jan 1, 1997.

Harvard. (2021). https://www.hsph.harvard.edu/nutritionsource/superfoods/. Retrieved November 3, 2021.

Hulkower, R. (2016). The history of the Hippocratic Oath: outdated, inauthentic, and yet still relevant. *Einstein Journal of Biology and Medicine, 25*(1), 41–44.

Khong, N. M., Yusoff, F. M., Jamilah, B., Basri, M., Maznah, I., Chan, K. W., & Nishiwaka, J. (2016). Nutritional composition and total collagen content of three commercially important edible jellyfish. *Food Chemistry, 196*, 953–960.

Kotecha, P. V. (2008). Micronutrient malnutrition in India: Let us say "no" to it now. *Indian Journal of Community Medicine: Official Publication of Indian Association of Preventive & Social Medicine, 33*(1), 9.

Kutala, V. K., Parinandi, N. L., Khan, M., Iyyapu, K. M., & Kuppusamy, P. (2008). Spirulina-a blue-green alga with novel therapeutic actions. *Phytopharmacology and Therapeutic Values, IV*, 127–151.

Lewis, J. (2020). Merck manual: Consumer version retrieved March 11, 2021 from: https://www.merckmanuals.com/home/hormonal-and-metabolic-disorders/electrolyte-balance/overview-of-sodiums-role-in-the-body

Madihassan, S. (1984). Outline of the beginning of alchemy and its antecedents. *The American Journal of Chinese Medicine, 12*, 32–42.

Mintz, S. W. (1986). *Sweetness and power: The place of sugar in modern history*. Penguin.

Mozaffarian, D., Rosenberg, I., & Uauy, R. (2018). History of modern nutrition science—Implications for current research, dietary guidelines, and food policy. *BMJ, 361*.

Nadolu, D., & Nadolu, B. (2019). About immortality: A socio-anthropological approach

Vandendriessche, F. (2008). Meat products in the past, today and in the future. *Meat Science, 78*(1–2), 104–113.

Verma, A. K. (2016). Evolution, merits and demerits of five kingdom system. *Flora and Fauna, 22*(1), 76–78.

Chapter 2
Avocados

Jeffrey P. Miller

2.1 Cultural History

The avocado originated in the temperate forests of central Mexico during the late Pleistocene epoch and did not spread far from its native roots until humans arrived in the Americas and began planting it in various places in Mesoamerica and the northern area of South America as they travelled and traded. The Spanish invaders of the New World encountered the avocado almost immediately upon arrival and were intrigued. It was totally unlike any food they had experienced in the Old World and descriptions of the fruit and tree were common in traveler accounts of the area in the sixteenth and seventeenth centuries (Silva & Ledesma, 2014). While avocados were grown in Spain as early as the sixteenth century (South African Avocado Grower's Yearbook, 1987) and were grown in Florida by the 1830s (Miller, 2020) they remained a novelty food outside Mesoamerica and the Caribbean until well into the twentieth century.

American growers of the avocado formed the California Avocado Association (initially named the California Ahuacate Association) in 1915 and assiduously promoted the fruit thereafter (Shepherd & Bender, 2002). The dominant avocado cultivar in global commerce is the Hass. The Hass avocado was first discovered in the orchard of Rudolf Hass in La Habra Heights, California in 1926 (Bost et al., 2013). The Hass avocado was the first tree to receive a plant patent (Plant Patent #139) in United States. While the Hass quickly became the dominant cultivar in American and global commerce, the patent was widely evaded by orchardists and Hass was said to have made less than $5000 on his patent in his lifetime (Miller, 2020).

Avocados began to impress themselves on the American psyche during the 1970s as California Cuisine, sushi, and guacamole became consumer favorites. American

J. P. Miller (✉)
Colorado State University, Fort Collins, CO, USA
e-mail: Jeffrey.miller@colostate.edu

© The Author(s), under exclusive license to Springer Nature Switzerland AG 2022
J. P. Miller, C. Van Buiten (eds.), *Superfoods*, Food and Health,
https://doi.org/10.1007/978-3-030-93240-4_2

consumption of avocados exploded after a series of advertisements promoting gua-camole appeared during the 1992 Super Bowl. The practice of eating avocado on toast is not new. Recipes in American media featuring the combination of avocado and toast go back at least one hundred years. The current vogue for avocado toast is attributed to Chef Bill Grainger of Melbourne, Australia. Grainger was looking for a high-priced item to boost breakfast profits at his café and hit upon avocado toast. According to Time magazine, in 2017, Americans spent nearly a million dollars a month on avocado toast at an average price of over six dollars per slice.

2.2   Nutritional Research on Avocado Consumption

Avocado Nutrition Avocados contain significant quantities of nutrients, including the minerals potassium, phosphorus, copper, calcium, and magnesium. They also contain a number of the B-complex vitamins such as niacin, pyroxidine, riboflavin, thiamin, and biotin. Avocados also have relatively high levels of vitamins C, E, & K. Avocados are one of the few foods that contain significant levels of both Vitamin C and Vitamin E in the same fruit (Dreher & Davenport, 2013). Avocados are rich in the unsaturated fatty acids lineoleic acid and palmitoleic acid. They also contain acetogenins, phytostanols, chlorophylls, carotenoids and alpha, beta, & gamma tocopherols. Avocados are significant sources of phytosterols (Duester, 2001). Phytosterols are natural, fat-like compounds with a structure that is similar to cho-lesterol. According to nutrition information provided by the Canadian government, natural plant sterols can help lower blood cholesterol, decrease the risk of certain cancers, and enhance immune systems (Patterson, 2006). The US Food & Drug Administration has approved package claims for plant sterol esters that allow manu-facturers to claim consumption of products enhanced with them can reduce the risk of heart disease (US Food & Drug Administration, 2020).

Though avocados have an unctuous mouthfeel due their relatively high fat con-tent, they are considered to have a medium energy density due to their high water content (as much as 80%) and high level of dietary fiber (Fulgoni et al., 2013.) Oil represents the largest energy constituent in avocados. The oil in avocados is mostly of the monounsaturated fatty acid type (MUFA), 66% on average, such as palmi-toleic and oleic acids and polyunsaturated fatty acids (PUFA), 15% on average, such as linoleic and linolenic acid (Mendez-Zuniga et al., 2019). Regular intake of MUFAs and PUFAs is associated with decreased incidence of cardiovascular dis-ease due to their ability to aid in the lowering of total serum cholesterol and low density lipoproteins (Mendez-Zuniga et al., 2019). Research studies reviewed by Mahmassani et al. (2018) showed that avocado intake can increase serum HDL concentrations. In the studies reviewed by Mahmassani et al. (2018) avocado sup-plementation was given at the level of 135 to 250 g per meal. The types of oil in the avocado, especially those of the MUFA type, help to increase the bioavailability of carotenoids from foods that are consumed at the same meal as the avocado (Fulgoni et al., 2013). Avocados have the highest lipophilic anti-oxidant capacity from vegetative food sources (Dreher & Davenport, 2013).

A medium-sized Hass avocado (weight 136 g) contains ~9.2 g of dietary fiber of which 70% is insoluble and 30% soluble (Henning et al., 2019). Dietary fiber makes up nearly 80% of the carbohydrate in an average avocado (Mahmsanni et al., 2018). The high level of dietary fiber combined with the relatively high level of fat in the fruit can reduce feelings of hunger and increase post-prandial satiety. Research by Wein et al. (2013) reported that participants who ate one-half of an average sized avocado with their luncheon meal reported increased satiation and reduced self-reported hunger.

While the avocado is technically a fruit, specifically a berry, it displays few of the sensory qualities most consumers associate with a food being a fruit. It is not sweet, it does not have the acidic component associated with most fruits, and it is relatively high in fat and protein (Miller, 2020). Unlike most fruits, avocados have negligible levels of glucose, fructose, and sucrose. Avocados do have high levels of seven carbon-atom sugars including D-mannoheptulose (MH). (Ramos-Aguilar et al., 2019). D-mannoheptulose and its reduced form, perseitol, are present at a level of ~4 g. in an average sized fruit. These forms of sugar don't behave in the body like the more common forms of fruit sugars (glucose, sucrose, fructose) and are considered more of a phytochemical than a dietary sugar. As a result, the glycemic load of avocados is nearly zero (Dreher & Davenport, 2013).

Avocados are one of the few fruits in the human diet with both water-soluble and fat-soluble components (Ramos-Aguilar et al., 2019). An average-sized avocado (~136 g) has a nutrient and phytochemical profile similar to 42.5 g of almonds, pistachios, or walnuts (Dreher & Davenport, 2013). Affects attributed to avocado consumption include reduction of oxidative stress and lipid oxidation, a decrease in lipoprotein lipase activity, the reduction of fat deposition in adipose tissue and reductions in cholesterol & triglycerides (Ramos-Aguilar et al., 2019).

Avocado pulp is a source of carotenoids. Carotenoids are red, orange, and yellow pigments that give color to vegetables like carrots and ripe tomatoes. Carotenoids are not synthesized in the human body, so they must come from dietary sources. Carotenoids are fat-soluble and absorbed better by the body when they are consumed with a dietary fat in the same meal. This makes avocados a useful food for carotenoid delivery. Carotenoids are also absorbed better when the food containing them is chopped, pureed, or similarly prepared. Carotenoids act as antioxidants in human cells (Pauling Center).

There are two primary types of carotenoids: xanthophylls and carotenes. The primary carotenoids in avocados are of the xanthophyll group, carotenoids that are oxygen-containing fat-soluble anti-oxidants (Dreher & Davenport, 2013). Avocado pulp is a good source of the carotenoids lutein, zeazanthin, and beta carotene (Mendez-Zuniga et al., 2019). Lutein is the most abundant carotenoid in avocado pulp (Ramos-Aguilar et al., 2019). The biovailability of lutein from avocados is higher than almost any other fruit or vegetable and the pigments in the skin and pulp contain high levels of various phytochemicals (Miller, 2020). It should be noted that the concentration of carotenoids is higher in the peel of the avocado than in the pulp. The primary avocado in global trade is the Hass, a cultivar with an inedible peel.

The primary reason that the Hass is such a popular cultivar among growers is the fact that it can be shipped green and ripened by the consumer with little-to-no loss of eating quality. A secondary reason for this popularity is the fact that the fruit can remain on the tree for many weeks after it attains maturity. This is a useful trait for a fruit that is still largely harvested by hand. Carotenoid levels tend to increase the longer the fruit hangs on the tree. Fruits harvested later after maturation tend to have less desirable sensory characteristics including being rubbery and/or stringy. Fruits with these characteristics often go to food processors who make them into guacamole or press them into oil. As a result, these secondary food products may have a stronger nutritional profile than the fresh fruit.

2.3 Related Science Topics

As noted earlier, the Hass cultivar dominates global commerce in avocados and has an inedible peel. The bulk of nutritional research has been done on the Hass cultivar due to support from the American avocado industry which overwhelmingly grows the Hass cultivar. There are cultivars with what is called "paper skin" which are commonly consumed in Mesoamerican cultures and the skin is consumed along with the pulp (Ramos-Aguilar et al., 2019). These cultivars, often referred to as heritage varieties, come from a family known collectively known as Drymifolia. The high level of anti-oxidants in the peel of Drymifolia suggest that there is benefit in preserving as wide a variety of subspecies as possible (Coralles-Garcia et al., 2019). Research by Coralles-Garcia et al. (2019) also suggests that some of these heritage varieties may be richer in MUFAs and PUFAs than the Hass cultivar.

Research on avocado-soy unsaponifiables (ASU) suggests that these vegetable extracts, which are a combination of approximately one-third avocado oil and two-thirds soybean oil may help in the palliative treatment of osteoarthritis. Research by Christiansen et al. (2015) showed a reduction of joint pain and stiffness when patients were treated with ASU. This may reduce the need for analgesic pain medicines in patients with osteoarthritis.

While research is preliminary, research by Pham et al. (2020) suggests that an enhanced extract from functional avocado oil named DKB 122 has otoprotective effects that can protect ear hair cells from the damage caused by aminoglycoside antibiotics. Use of these antibiotics is one of the leading causes of Sensorineural hearing loss (SNHL), a common affliction worldwide (Nam et al., 2019).

Parts of the avocado other than pulp are popular in homeopathic remedies. The highest concentration of phenolic compounds is in the pit rather than the pulp (Miller, 2020). Ground pits have astringent qualities and are used in homeopathic cures where this property is desirable. Ground pits are also used as a larvicide and fungicide in some places (Lara-Marquez et al., 2020).

2.4 Social Issues in Avocado Production and Distribution

While avocados have what is called "unicorn status" nutritionally, that is they are a fatty food that is good for you and may even help you lose weight; that status does not extend to other qualities of avocados and their production. One problematic area in avocado production is water usage. Virtually everywhere avocados are grown in the world, they are an irrigated crop. In places like their home state of Michoacán, Mexico the extra water required to grow avocados commercially is not wildly extravagant. But even in Michoacán, where the fruit is native, growers use over 30 gallons of irrigation water to grow one pound of avocados. In places like Chile and parts of Australian where avocados grow well, but the climate is very dry, it takes nearly 100 gallons of irrigation water to produce a pound of avocados (Mother Jones, 2014).

Mexico is the largest grower and exporter of avocados globally, accounting for more than 30% of world consumption (Araujo et al., 2018). Given the periodic crackdowns on criminal gangs in Mexico by the national government, these gangs, who often are referred to as *narcotraficantes,* are turning to licit industries to maintain cashflows and profitability. The avocado industries in the states of Michoacan and Jalisco, the largest producers of avocados in the world, have been targeted by the *narcotraficantes* as a source of licit revenues (Dehgan, 2019). These groups control some orchards and processors directly and charge a "tax" on other growers in the region (Miller, 2020). A single gang, the *Caballeros Templarios* are said to control 10% of avocado production in the two states and make as much as 100 million dollars a year from these activities and they are just one of the gangs operating in the prime avocado growing areas in Mexico (Frazier, 2018).

As noted above, the largest center of world avocado production is in central Mexico. This area is also home to the oyamel fir tree, a critical habitat for overwintering Monarch butterflies. Due to illegal logging and unlicensed avocado orcharding, this habit is shrinking causing habitat loss for the monarch butterfly. In addition, avocado trees capture four to five times the amount of water that oyamel firs do, leaving less to recharge groundwater while capturing only a quarter of the carbon dioxide of oyamel firs (Global Forest Watch, 2019).

2.5 Recipes

Avocado, Crab, and Asparagus Louis *–this dish is the definition of elegance and is very easy to make. Make sure you pick the crab well for shell fragments, but try not to break up the meat too much; big lumps of crabmeat are very impressive.*

1 lb. asparagus – trimmed, steamed, chilled
1 lb. cooked lump crab meat – picked for shell fragments
1 or 2 large avocados – peeled and diced immediately before serving
1 or 2 large eggs – hard cooked, peeled and chopped
To taste – salt and pepper

Louis Sauce:

>   2 cups mayonnaise
>   1 cup Heinz chili sauce
>   Juice of one lime
>   2 Tbsp grated prepared horseradish
>   1/eighth tsp. cayenne pepper
>   (optional: one quarter of a medium sweet onion, like a Vidalia – grated, keep
>   the juice)

Start by making the Louis sauce and putting it in the refrigerator to chill.

Place the asparagus spears on the plate. Sprinkle the crab over the asparagus spears. Dress with the Louis sauce to taste. Top with the avocado cubes. Sprinkle the chopped egg over the top and season with salt and pepper if desired.

Avocado Chicken Tortilla Soup – *one of the classic dishes of Mexico and Central America. The avocado adds a cooling note to the warm broth. Using premade broth and canned or rotisserie chicken, this is truly a meal in minutes.*

32 ounces chicken broth – homemade or packaged
12 to 14 ounces chicken meat (boneless breast or boneless thigh)– can be fresh
    cooked, canned, or rotisserie chicken
To taste – black pepper, cumin, coriander, chili powder (start with about ¼ teaspoon
    of each and adjust from there.)
1 or 2 avocados, peeled and diced just before serving
Tortilla chips for garnish

Mix together your broth and chicken meat and spices and bring to a boil. Reduce heat to low and simmer for about 15 minutes. Taste your broth and adjust your seasonings. If you used homemade broth, you may want to add salt here. If using prepackaged broth, it should be salty enough already.

Avocado Toast – *you probably don't really need a recipe for this, but try one of the variations.*

A slice of your favorite bread, well toasted.
About a half an avocado mashed on top.
Always start with a sprinkle of salt and black pepper. Then get creative with the toppings. The classic is a dash of red pepper flakes, but my personal favorite is white anchovy fillet. If you are feeling rich, try Spanish jamon or smoked salmon. Feeling daring? Try a schmeer of goat yogurt and a sprinkle of zaatar spice. One of the greatest variations is toasted sunflower seeds and English cucumber sliced paper thin.

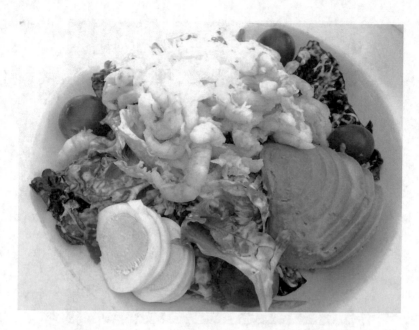

Shrimp Louis Salad. (Neeta Lind, CC BY 2.0 <https://creativecommons.org/licenses/by/2.0>, via Wikimedia Commons)

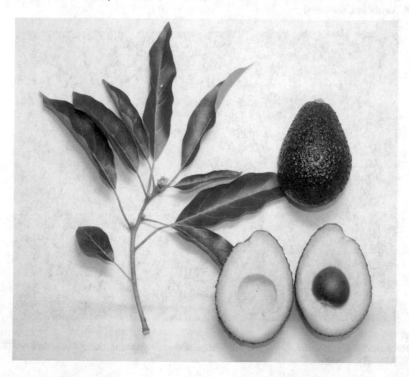

Avocado Tree and Fruit. (Edrean, CC BY-SA 3.0 <https://creativecommons.org/licenses/by-sa/3.0>, via Wikimedia Commons)

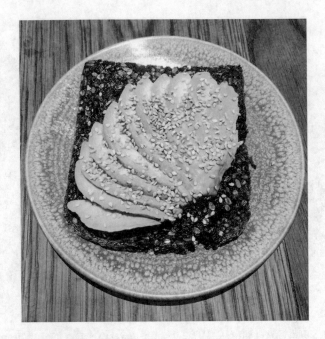

Avocado Toast. (Jami430, CC BY-SA 4.0 <https://creativecommons.org/licenses/by-sa/4.0>, via Wikimedia Commons)

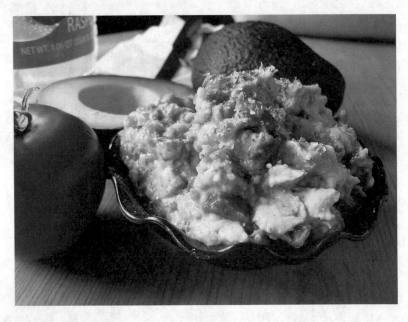

Guacamole. (stu_spivack, CC BY-SA 2.0 <https://creativecommons.org/licenses/by-sa/2.0>, via Wikimedia Commons)

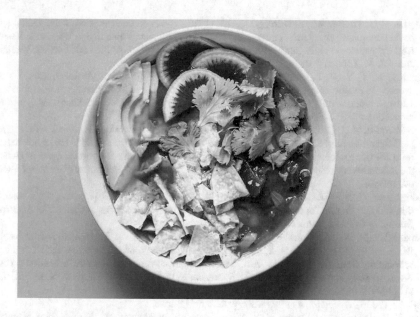

Avocado Tortilla Soup. (spurekar, CC BY 2.0 <https://creativecommons.org/licenses/by/2.0>, via Wikimedia Commons)

References

Araújo, R. G., Rodriguez-Jasso, R. M., Ruiz, H. A., Pintado, M. M. E., & Aguilar, C. N. (2018). Avocado byproducts: Nutritional and functional properties. *Trends in Food Science and Technology, 80*, 51–60. https://doi.org/10.1016/j.tifs.2018.07.027

Bost, J. B., Smith, N. J. H., & Crane, J. H. (2013). *History, distribution and uses. The avocado: Botany, production and uses* (2nd ed., pp. 10–30). Centre for Agriculture and Biosciences International.

Christiansen, B. A., et al. (2015). Management of osteoarthritis with avocado/soybean unsaponifiables. *Cartilage, 6*(1), 30–44. https://doi.org/10.1177/1947603514554992

Corrales-García, J. E., del Rosario García-Mateos, M., Martínez-López, E., Barrientos-Priego, A. F., Ybarra-Moncada, M. C., Ibarra-Estrada, E., Méndez-Zúñiga, S. M., & Becerra-Morales, D. (2019). Anthocyanin and oil contents, fatty acids profiles and antioxidant activity of Mexican landrace avocado fruits. *Plant Foods for Human Nutrition, 74*(2), 210–215.

Dehghan, S. (2019). *Are Mexican avocados the world's new conflict commodity?* The Guardian: Global Development. 30 December.

Dreher, M. L., & Davenport, A. J. (2013). Hass avocado composition and potential health effects. *Critical Reviews in Food Science and Nutrition, 53*(7), 738–750.

Duester, K. C. (2001). Avocado fruit is a rich source of beta-sitosterol. *Journal of the Academy of Nutrition and Dietetics, 101*(4), 404.

Forests Falling Fast to Make Way for Mexican Avocado. Global Forest Watch, 2019, March 20. Retrieved March 1, 2021.

Frazier, B. (2018). *Blood avocados: Cracking down on the cartels.* Brown Political Review. 2018, April 18. Retrieved March 1, 2021.

Fulgoni, V. L., Dreher, M., & Davenport, A. J. (2013). Avocado consumption is associated with better diet quality and nutrient intake, and lower metabolic syndrome risk in US adults: Results from the National Health and Nutrition Examination Survey (NHANES) 2001–2008. *Nutrition Journal, 12*, 1. https://doi.org/10.1186/1475-2891-12-1

Henning, S. M., Yang, J., Woo, S. L., Lee, R.-P., Huang, J., Rasmusen, A., et al. (2019). Hass avocado inclusion in a weight-loss diet supported weight loss and altered gut microbiota: A 12-week randomized, parallel-controlled trial. *Current Developments in Nutrition, 3*, nzz068. https://doi.org/10.1093/cdn/nzz068

Lara-Marquez, M., Baez-Magana, M., Raymundo-Ramos, C., Spagnuolo, P. A., Macias-Rodriguez, L., Salgado-Garciglia, R., Ochoa-Zarzosa, A., & Lopez-Meza, J. E. (2020). Lipid-rich extract from Mexican avocado (Persea americana var. drymifolia) induces apoptosis and modulates the inflammatory response in Caco-2 human colon cancer cells. *Journal of Functional Foods, 64*, 103658.

Mahmassani, H. A., Avendano, E. E., Raman, G., & Johnson, E. J. (2018). Avocado consumption and risk factors for heart disease: A systematic review and meta-analysis. *The American Journal of Clinical Nutrition, 107*(4), 523–536.

Méndez-Zúñiga, S. M., Corrales-García, J. E., Gutiérrez-Grijalva, E. P., García-Mateos, R., Pérez-Rubio, V., & Heredia, J. B. (2019). Fatty acid profile, total carotenoids, and free radical-scavenging from the lipophilic fractions of 12 native Mexican avocado accessions. *Plant Foods for Human Nutrition (Dordrecht, Netherlands), 74*(4), 501–507. https://doi.org/10.1007/s11130-019-00766-2

Miller, J. (2020). *Avocado: A global history*. Reaktion Books.

Nam, Y. H., Rodriguez, I., Jeong, S. Y., Pham, T. N. M., Nuankaew, W., Kim, Y. H., Castañeda, R., Jeong, S. Y., Park, M. S., Lee, K. W., & Lee, J. S. (2019). Avocado oil extract modulates auditory hair cell function through the regulation of amino acid biosynthesis genes. *Nutrients, 11*(1), 113.

Patterson, C.A. (July 2006). "Phytosterols and stanols: Topic 10075E" (PDF). Agriculture and Agri-Food Canada, Government of Canada. Retrieved February 19, 2021.

Pham, T. N. M., Jeong, S. Y., Kim, D. H., Park, Y. H., Lee, J. S., Lee, K. W., Moon, I. S., Choung, S. Y., Kim, S. H., Kang, T. H., & Jeong, K. W. (2020). Protective mechanisms of avocado oil extract against ototoxicity. *Nutrients, 12*(4), 947.

Philpott, T. (2014). 'It Takes HOW Much Water to Grow an Avocado?', *Mother Jones,* 2014, October 1, 2014. Retrieved March 1, 2021.

Ramos-Aguilar, A. L., Ornelas-Paz, J., Tapia-Vargas, L. M., Ruiz-Cruz, S., Gardea-Béjar, A. A., Yahia, E. M., de Jesús Ornelas-Paz, J., Pérez-Martínez, J. D., Rios-Velasco, C., & Ibarra-Junquera, V. (2019). The importance of the bioactive compounds of avocado fruit (Persea americana Mill) on human health. *Biotecnia, 21*(3), 154–162.

Shepherd, J., & Bender, G. (2002). A history of the avocado industry in California. *California Avocado Society 2001 Yearbook,85*.

Silva, T. A., & Ledesma, N. (2014). Avocado history, biodiversity and production. In *Sustainable horticultural systems* (pp. 157–205). Springer.

South African Avocado Growers' Association Yearbook 1987. 10:27–28. Proceedings of the First World Avocado Congress – Accessed 28 Jan 2021.

US Food & Drug Administration. (2020). CFR – Title 21. https://www.accessdata.fda.gov/scripts/cdrh/cfdocs/cfcfr/CFRSearch.cfm?fr=101.83. Retrieved 19 Feb 2021.

Wein, M., Haddad, E., Oda, K., & Sabate, J. (2013). A randomized 3x3 crossover study to evaluate the effect of Hass avocado intake on post-ingestive satiety, glucose and insulin levels, and subsequent energy intake in overweight adults. *Nutrition Journal, 12*, 155.

Chapter 3
Bush Berries

Sarah A. Johnson and Emily K. Woolf

3.1 A Cultural History of Bush Berries

Bush berries, such as aronia berries (also known as chokeberries), blackberries, blueberries, currants, elderberries, and raspberries, are berries that grow on bushes. For centuries, they have been used for foods, medicines, herbal remedies, dyes and food colorants, and cosmetics. Most bush berries were cultivated and domesticated in the early twentieth century, though blackberries (Fig. 3.1) were cultivated in the nineteenth century, and red raspberries as early as the fourth century by Romans (Charlebois, 2007; Clark & Finn, 2014; Dale et al., 1993; Mainland, 2012; Shahin et al., 2019). Hippocrates (460–375 BC) recommended soaking blackberry stems and leaves in white wine to help with childbirth (Ferlemi & Lamari, 2016). Blackberries are now grown in the United States (US) primarily in Oregon, Central America, and Europe (Clark & Finn, 2014), while red raspberries are also grown in the US (primarily in Oregon, Washington, and California), as well as in Europe (primarily Serbia and Poland), and Chile (Strik, 2007). Interestingly, blackberries and raspberries are also referred to as caneberries, as their bushes produce woody, hard stems that resemble canes (Fernandez et al., 2016).

Native to North America, aronia berries were used by Forest Pottawatomi Native Americans to make teas for treating colds and were used in food dishes. In the twentieth century they were introduced to eastern Europe and the Soviet Union for use in food products, wines, and food colorants (Kokotkiewicz et al., 2010). Today, Poland produces the majority of aronia berries (NDSU Carrington Research Extension Center).

S. A. Johnson (✉) · E. K. Woolf
Department of Food Science and Human Nutrition, Colorado State University,
Fort Collins, CO, USA
e-mail: Sarah.Johnson@colostate.edu; Emily.Woolf@colostate.edu

© The Author(s), under exclusive license to Springer Nature Switzerland AG 2022
J. P. Miller, C. Van Buiten (eds.), *Superfoods*, Food and Health,
https://doi.org/10.1007/978-3-030-93240-4_3

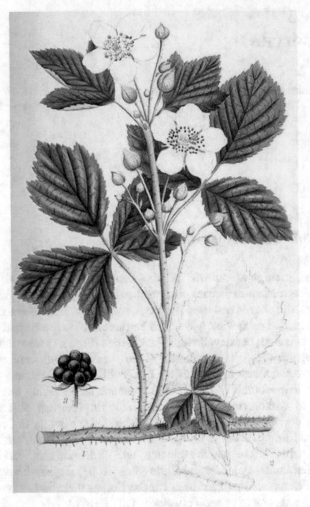

Fig. 3.1 Blackberry plant. Carl Axel Magnus Lindman, Public domain, via Wikimedia Commons

Blueberries were domesticated in the US by Frederick Vernon Coville, who began to cultivate them in 1906 by designing and implementing his own research on how to grow blueberries for sell and trade instead of being reliant on wild berries. He was interested in blueberries for their ability to uphold rough treatment, such as shipment, compared to other berries, making them readily available to the market in first-class condition (Mainland, 2012). Highbush blueberries are the predominant modern-day cultivars, with production highest in North America, followed by South America, Europe, Asian and Pacific regions, and Africa (Villata & Council, 2012). Lowbush wild blueberries are native to North America and grow in the harsh northern climates of Maine in the US and eastern Canada (Wild Blueberries of North America).

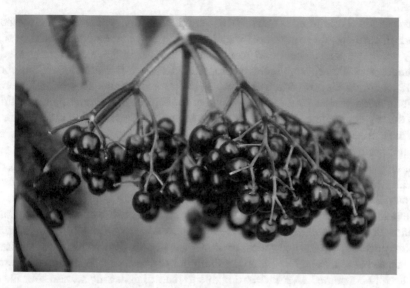

Fig. 3.2 Ripe elderberries growing by the Roman wall at Calleva Atrebatum. Elderberries can be used in a number of ways, including making elderberry wine. Stephen McKay/Elderberries, via Wikimedia coomons

In the twentieth century, elderberries were cultivated in northern America, but are now grown in North America, Europe, northern Africa, and parts of Asia. They have been used in several countries to keep evil spirits away (Charlebois, 2007). Black elderberries (Fig. 3.2) are known as European elderberries whereas red elderberries are known as American elderberries and are primarily grown on the northwestern coast in Oregon, Washington, and northern California (Charlebois, 2007).

There are several different types of currants (e.g. black, white, golden, ornamental, and red) grown in Eastern European countries such as Russia and Poland, as well as Germany, Great Britain, Scandinavia, and New Zealand. Currants are native to North America but were also imported into North America by early trade ships. In the late 1800s, it was determined that a fungus responsible for White Pine Blister Rust was also being imported, and the disease was reported in White Pine trees throughout the Northeast by 1911. This led to a federal ban against importation and cultivation of currants until 1966, but many states continued the ban. Thus, currants have not been widely produced in the US (Cortez & Gonzalez De Mejia, 2019; Hummer & Barney, 2002; UMass-Extension, 2012).

Bush berries have been used for their purported and substantiated medicinal properties. In addition to using the berries, other parts of the plants have been used as well. For example, the berries and their leaves have been used to combat colds, inflammation, urinary tract infections, diabetes, diarrhea, sore throat, and/or ocular dysfunction by Native Americans and other populations (Ferlemi & Lamari, 2016). Blackberry juice has been used fight against colitis (Verma et al., 2014), while raspberry leaves are often used to reduce anemia, fatigue and petulance during menstruation (Ferlemi & Lamari, 2016). Aronia berry tea was traditionally used to ward off cold and flu symptoms (Shahin et al., 2019), and elderberries have similarly and more lately been used to fight against fever and are commonly used in lozenges and dietary supplements promoted for immune function (Charlebois, 2007; Sidor & Gramza-Michałowska, 2015). Other unique uses of elderberries include using berries as a laxative, flowers for topical anti-inflammatory actions, and the leaves and inner bark of the bush as a diuretic. The impact of elderberries on diarrhea, nasal congestion, and respiration has been credited to its tannins and viburnic acid content (Charlebois, 2007). Lastly, blackberry leaves have been used as a tonic and mouthwash for treating thrush, gum inflammation, sore throat, and mouth ulcers, and are chewed to strengthen gums and cure thrush (Ferlemi & Lamari, 2016).

In addition to the consumption of fresh and frozen bush berries, they have also been used by the food industry to make products such as food colorants, jams and jellies, juices, syrups, sauces, teas, beers, wines, liquors (Zhao, 2007). Elderberries are somewhat toxic and require processing prior to consumption, and aronia berries are usually consumed after processing due to their high astringent and sour flavors (Shahin et al., 2019). Bush berries are commonly used in cosmetic products such as soaps and shampoos, and body lotions, creams, and balms, largely due to their antioxidant and anti-inflammatory properties (Kokotkiewicz et al., 2010; Piazza et al., 2020; Verma et al., 2014).

3.2 Current State of Nutritional Research and Health Claims for Bush Berries

Bush berries contain a diverse range of nutrients including vitamins, minerals, and dietary fiber (Table 3.1). Some bush berries contain notable amounts of certain vitamins and minerals. For instance, blueberries are particularly rich in manganese, with a 100 gram portion of fresh berries providing up to 500 micrograms or 25% of the Dietary Reference Intake (DRI), though other berry types such as blackberries and raspberries are high in the mineral as well. Blackberries and blueberries are rich sources of vitamin K. Black currants are particularly high in vitamin C relative to other bush berries, with 100 g of the fresh berry providing more than the DRI (Cortez & Gonzalez De Mejia, 2019).

Bush berries are also rich in non-nutrient compounds referred to as phytochemicals (i.e. plant chemicals) or bioactive compounds due to their biological activity in animals and humans. Phytochemicals present in berries are called polyphenols, which are secondary plant metabolites containing one or more phenolic groups. Polyphenols can be classified as flavonoids (e.g. anthocyanins, flavonols, flavan-3-ols) or non-flavonoids (e.g. phenolic acids, stilbenes, tannins). Environmental factors such as plant genotype, growing conditions, environmental factors including the geographic growing region and climate, ripeness, and post-harvest factors like storage conditions can affect the nutritional quality and concentrations of

Table 3.1 Nutritional composition of select bush berries (per 100 g fresh berries)

	Blueberry (fresh)	Blackcurrant (fresh)	Raspberry (fresh)	Elderberry (fresh)	Blackberry (fresh)
Energy (kcal)	57	63	52	73	43
Protein (g)	0.7	1.4	1.2	0.7	1.4
Lipid (g)	0.33	0.41	0.65	0.50	0.49
Carbohydrate (g)	14.49	15.38	11.94	18.40	9.61
Total fiber (g)	2.4	ND	6.5	7.0	5.3
Total sugars (g)	9.96	ND	4.42	ND	4.88
Iron (mg)	0.28	1.54	0.69	1.60	0.62
Sodium (mg)	1	2	1	6	1
Manganese (mg)	0.33	0.26	0.67	ND	ND
Copper (mg)	0.06	0.09	0.09	0.06	0.17
Zinc (mg)	0.16	0.27	0.42	0.11	0.53
Calcium (mg)	6	55	25	38	29
Phosphorus (mg)	12	59	29	39	22
Potassium (mg)	77	322	151	280	162
Magnesium (mg)	6	24	22	5	20
Selenium (µg)	0.1	ND	0.2	0.6	0.4
Vitamin C (mg)	9.7	181.0	26.2	36.0	21.0
Thiamin (mg)	0.04	0.05	0.03	0.07	0.02
Riboflavin (mg)	0.04	0.05	0.04	0.06	0.03
Niacin (mg)	0.42	0.30	0.60	0.5	0.65
Pantothenic acid (mg)	0.12	0.4	0.33	0.14	ND
Vitamin B6 (mg)	0.05	0.07	0.06	0.23	0.03
Folate (µg)	6	ND	21	6	25
Vitamin B12 (mg)	0	0	0	0	0
Vitamin A (µg)	3	12	2	30	11
Vitamin E, total (mg)	0.57	1.00	0.87	ND	1.17
Choline (mg)	6.0	ND	12.3	ND	8.5
Carotene, beta (µg)	32	ND	12	ND	128
Carotene, alpha (µg)	0	ND	16	ND	0
Lutein + zeaxanthin (µg)	80	ND	136	ND	118
Vitamin K (µg)	19.3	ND	7.8	ND	19.8

ND = No data available
Source: FoodData Central (usda.gov)

polyphenols in berries, which will determine the amount of any given nutrient or polyphenol present and consumed.

There are numerous purported health claims for bush berries (Table 3.2). However, no health claims have been approved by the US Food and Drug Administration (FDA). The exception is for cranberries, which are not technically

Table 3.2 Possible health properties of bush berries

Berries	Prominent phytochemicals	Possible health properties	References
Blueberry	Anthocyanins (60% of total polyphenolic compounds); proanthocyanidins; flavonols; hydroxycinnamic acid esters (chlorogenic acid)	Antioxidant; cardiovascular health; protects against weight gain; improves blood lipids; positive effects on blood pressure and arterial stiffness; reduces risk for type 2 diabetes mellitus; neuroprotection; improves cognition; & beneficial for vision and eye health	Wilhelmina et al. (2020) and Kalt et al. (2020)
Blackcurrant	Anthocyanins; anthocyanidins	Antioxidant; anti-inflammatory; hypocholesterolemia; positive effects on low-density lipoprotein-cholesterol and glucose; increase fat oxidation; biosynthesis of collagen and peptide production	Cortez and Gonzalez de Mejia (2019) Barik et al. (2020)
Aronia berry	Procyanidins (66% of total phenol content); anthocyanins (25% of total phenol content); chlorogenic acid; neochlorogenic acid	Decrease blood pressure and weight gain; anti-inflammatory; improves cognition; antioxidant; positive effects on blood glucose and insulin; cardioprotective; improves blood lipids	King and Bolling (2020)
Raspberry	Ellagitannins; anthocyanins	Reduce risk for diabetes mellitus, obesity, and cardiovascular disease; antioxidant; anti-inflammatory; positive effects on endothelial function; improves diabetic symptoms; & protective against DNA damage in cells	Singh et al. (n.d.) and Gao et al. (2018)
Elderberry	Phenolic acids; tannins; anthocyanins; saponins	Antioxidant; beneficial for blood pressure and blood lipids; protective against diabetes mellitus and obesity risk; antiviral; antibacterial; antifungal; anti-inflammatory; protection against UV radiation; laxative; & diuretic	Sidor and Gramza-Michałowska (2015) and Vujanović et al. (2020)
Blackberry	Anthocyanins; ellagic acid; ellagitannins; epi/catechin; proanthocyanidins	Anti-inflammatory; chemoprotective; neuroprotective; reduces insulin resistance and weight gain; cognitive function; benefits to bone density; cardioprotective	Robinson et al. (2020)

bush berries, but rather are low-growing, vining, woody perennial plants commonly found in bogs or marshes (Massachusetts Cranberries). The FDA allows cranberry supplement and juice products to use a qualified health claim on product labels and for marketing purposes, specifically with regard to reducing the risk of recurrent urinary tract infections in healthy women. The supplement serving size must contain 500 mg for use each day, while the juice serving size should be 8 ounces for use each day (FDA, 2020). Qualified health claims are supported by scientific evidence but do not meet the standards of rigorous scientific evidence for an authorized health claim (FDA, 2019).

Strong epidemiological evidence suggests that anthocyanin-rich berry consumption, particularly blueberries, is linked to a reduced risk for cardiovascular disease (Kalt et al., 2020; Speer et al., 2020). Pre-clinical and clinical studies have also shown that blueberry consumption can improve vascular function (Wood et al., 2019), which is significant given the role that vascular dysfunction plays in cardiovascular disease development (Johnson et al., 2019). However, their effects on other cardiovascular risk factors such as blood pressure and blood lipid profiles are less clearly established (Speer et al., 2020). Pre-clinical and clinical studies have also observed anti-cancer properties associated with various berry types and notably black raspberries, blackberries, and blueberries, with the greatest effects observed in cancers of the gastrointestinal tract and the breast (Kristo et al., 2016). Blueberries and blackcurrants (Fig. 3.3) can also prevent bone loss in animals, however these

Fig. 3.3 Ripening blackcurrant. Petr Kratochvil, CC0, via Wikimedia Commons

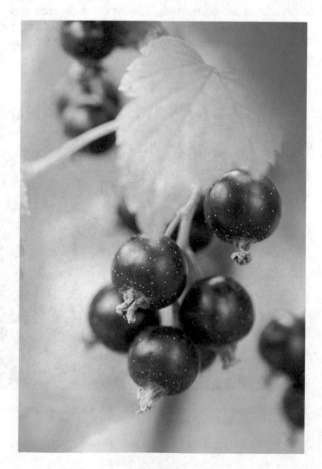

effects require confirmation in humans. (Devareddy et al., 2008; Li et al., 2014; Sakaki et al., 2018; Zhang et al., 2011, 2013; Zheng et al., 2016). Bush berries, particularly blueberries and aronia berries, appear to also serve a neurocognitive protective role in both animal and human studies (Ahles et al., 2020; Daskalova et al., 2019; Hein et al., 2019; Kalt et al., 2020; Lee et al., 2016). Examples of the health effects of bush berries, including those mentioned here, are listed in Table 3.2.

3.3   Science Behind Bush Berries

Among the polyphenols present in bush berries, anthocyanins are water-soluble pigmented compounds that accumulate within the vacuoles of the plant tissue. They are the most abundant and widely distributed class of flavonoids in red, blue, and/or purple pigmented berries. Their production is stimulated by light, and they are important in plant pollination, light absorption, and protection against ultraviolet light (UV) and cold stress (Mattioli et al., 2020; Rodriguez-Mateos et al., 2014). Certain berries such as blueberries, aronia berries (Fig. 3.4), blackcurrants, and elderberries are particularly known for their rich anthocyanin contents, though other bush berries contain anthocyanins as well. The types of anthocyanins present in bush berries differ among the berry types. For instance, redcurrants, elderberries,

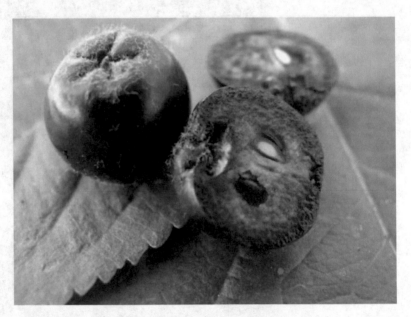

Fig. 3.4 Aronia berry. Healthshare, CC BY-SA 4.0 <https://creativecommons.org/licenses/by-sa/4.0>, via Wikimedia Commons

blackberries, and raspberries contain derivatives of cyanidin, while blueberries contain derivatives of multiple types of anthocyanins such as cyanidin, delphinidin, petunidin, and malvidin, and blackcurrants contain derivatives of cyanidin and delphinidin (Del Rio et al., 2010). Due to their complex chemical structure, anthocyanins are poorly bioavailable in the small intestine and must be metabolized to smaller compounds, such as phenolic acids, by the gut microbiota in the large intestine prior to their absorption and further metabolism by the liver. As such, the composition of the gut microbiota can influence the bioavailability of anthocyanins and thus the health effects of anthocyanin-rich berry consumption (Lavefve et al., 2020).

Flavan-3-ols and flavonols are among the other flavonoid compounds found in berries and range from simple monomers to complex oligomer and polymer compounds (i.e. oligomeric and polymeric proanthocyanidins known as condensed or non-hydrolyzable tannins) (Rodriguez-Mateos et al., 2014). Flavonols accumulate in the outer tissues of plants and their production is stimulated by light, while flavan-3-ols are found in the peels and seeds of berry fruits (de Pascual-Teresa et al., 2010; Manach et al., 2004). Flavan-3-ols and flavonols vary in their bioavailability depending on the degree of polymerization, among other factors, and thus some types can be absorbed within a few hours in the small intestine while others must be metabolized by the gut microbiota (de Pascual-Teresa et al., 2010).

Phenolic acids, especially hydroxycinnamic acids and hydroxybenzoic acids, are common phytochemicals in bush berries (Lavefve et al., 2020). They are aromatic compounds containing one phenolic ring and at least one organic carboxylic acid functionality (Kumar & Goel, 2019). These compounds can be absorbed early in the proximal gastrointestinal tract following berry consumption, likely contributing to many of their early acute health effects (about 1–2 hours following consumption). They are also absorbed in the colon following microbiota fermentation of more complex polyphenols (e.g. anthocyanins) and their resulting production, likely contributing to later acute health effects (about 6 hours after consumption) (Lavefve et al., 2020). Improvements in endothelial function have been observed at 1, 2, and 6 hours post-blueberry consumption (Wood et al., 2019).

Stilbenes are phenolic compounds comprised of two aromatic rings linked by a double bond, and can occur in berry fruits as monomers, dimers, and oligomers. Common stilbenes found in berry fruits include resveratrol, pterostilbene, and picetannol, which predominately accumulate in berry skins during development (Błaszczyk et al., 2019). Of the bush berries, blueberries (Fig. 3.5) are known for their stilbene contents, especially pterostilbene, which is a more potent and bioavailable analog of resveratrol, known for its various biological and health-promoting properties (Kim et al., 2020; Liu et al., 2020; Paredes-López et al., 2010).

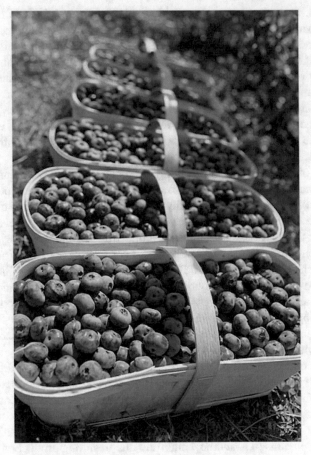

Fig. 3.5 Blueberries during the harvest season on a blueberry plantation in Québec, Canada. Healthshare, CC BY-SA 4.0, via Wikimedia Commons

3.4   Social Issues

Though bush berries have high nutritional quality and are increasingly well-known for their impacts on human health, they do have interactions with the environment and the global food system of note. For instance, global climate change including warming temperatures has impacted the growth patterns of wild blueberries in Maine and emerging research indicates a negative impact on plant performance. Though preliminary, this may extend to other bush berries and necessitates further research and development of methods for improving adaptation to climate change for farmers (Tasnim et al., 2020).

Another issue is that of marketing bush berries for consumption based on their health benefits. Many berry agricultural commodity boards, for example, provide financial support for academic research studies to evaluate the health effects of the specific food crop. The results of the studies are promoted and used for marketing purposes to increase consumption of the commodity. However, it has been suggested that the foundation of such research is misleading and raises questions about biases in the design, conduct, and interpretation of the research (Nestle, 2018), which is largely unfounded. Lastly, given the environmental impacts of food packaging waste, it is noteworthy that in 2020, several berry growers committed to using 100% recycle-ready packaging. The use of clamshell packaging is important to the industry as it minimizes product damage and contamination and therefore food waste (Nauseda, 2020).

Organophosphate pesticides, which are derivatives of phosphoric acid, have been used extensively in commercial and residential agriculture since the late 1970s. Organophosphate insecticides used in the wild blueberry industry include phosmet, azinphos-methyl, malathion, and diazinon to control blueberry maggot. Typically, the bulk of blueberries are individually quick frozen following a chlorinated wash. A recent study demonstrated that distilled water rinses reduced residual levels of insecticide by 30% and the addition of chlorine (100–200 ppm) resulted in a further 15% reduction (Hazen et al., 2004).

3.5 Recipe(s)

Blackberry Breakfast Bars *Ingredients:*

- 2 cups fresh or frozen blackberries or raspberries
- 2 tablespoons sugar
- 2 tablespoons water
- 1 tablespoon lemon juice
- 1/2 teaspoon ground cinnamon
- 1 cup all-purpose flour
- 1 cup quick cooking rolled oats
- 2/3 cup packed brown sugar
- 1/4 teaspoon ground cinnamon
- 1/8 teaspoon baking soda
- 1/2 cup margarine or butter melted

Instructions:

1. For filling, in a medium saucepan combine berries, sugar, water, lemon juice and ½ teaspoon cinnamon.
2. Bring to a boil.
3. Reduce heat. Simmer, uncovered, for about 8 minutes or till slightly thickened, stirring frequently.

4. Remove from heat.
5. In a mixing bowl stir together flour, oats, brown sugar, ¼ teaspoon cinnamon, and baking soda.
6. Stir in melted margarine or butter till thoroughly combined.
7. Set aside 1 cup of the oat mixture for topping. Press remaining oat mixture into an ungreased 9 × 9 × 2-inch pan. Bake in a 350-degree oven for 20 to 25 minutes.
8. Carefully spread filling on top of baked crust.
9. Sprinkle with reserved oat mixture.
10. Lightly press oat mixture into filling.
11. Bake in the 350-degree oven for 20 to 25 minutes more or till topping is set. Cool in pan on a wire rack.
12. Cut into bars. Makes 18

Source: North American Raspberry and Blackberry Association, https://www.raspberryblackberry.com/recipes/blackberry-breakfast-bars/

Savory Blueberry Pizza *Ingredients:*

- 1 pound pizza dough
- 1–1/2 cups grated mozzarella cheese, divided
- 1/2 cup crumbled gorgonzola cheese
- 4 ounces diced pancetta (can also use bacon or ham if pancetta is not available), cooked and drained
- 1/4 cup thinly sliced red onion
- 1 cup fresh blueberries
- 1/4 cup thinly sliced fresh basil
- Freshly ground black pepper

Instructions:

1. Preheat oven to 450 °F
2. Lightly flour a work surface
3. Pat and stretch dough into a 10 × 14-inch oval; place on a large baking sheet
4. With a fork, pierce dough in several places
5. Leaving a 1-inch border, sprinkle dough with half the mozzarella, the gorgonzola, pancetta and red onion
6. Bake until crust is golden brown, 12 to 14 minutes
7. Sprinkle blueberries and remaining mozzarella over pizza; bake until cheese is melted and crust is golden brown, about 2 minutes longer
8. Remove from oven; top with basil and pepper

Source: U.S. Highbush Blueberry Council, https://www.blueberrycouncil.org/blueberry-recipe/savory-blueberry-pizza/

References

Ahles, S., Stevens, Y. R., Joris, P. J., Vauzour, D., Adam, J., De Groot, E., & Plat, J. (2020). The effect of long-term Aronia melanocarpa extract supplementation on cognitive performance, mood, and vascular function: a randomized controlled trial in healthy, middle-aged individuals. *Nutrients, 12*, 2475.

Barik, S. K., Russell, W. R., Moar, K. M., Cruickshank, M., Scobbie, L., Duncan, G., & Hoggard, N. (2020). The anthocyanins in black currants regulate postprandial hyperglycaemia primarily by inhibiting α-glucosidase while other phenolics modulate salivary α-amylase, glucose uptake and sugar transporters. *The Journal of Nutritional Biochemistry, 78*, 108325.

Błaszczyk, A., Sady, S., & Sielicka, M. (2019). The stilbene profile in edible berries. *Phytochemistry Reviews, 18*, 37–67.

Charlebois, D. (2007). Elderberry as a medicinal plant. In *Issues in new crops and new uses* (pp. 284–292). ASHS Press.

Clark, J. R., & Finn, C. E. (2014). Blackberry cultivation in the world. *Revista Brasileira de Fruticultura, 36*, 46–57.

Cortez, R. E., & Gonzalez De Mejia, E. (2019). Blackcurrants (Ribes nigrum): A review on chemistry, processing, and health benefits. *Journal of Food Science, 84*, 2387–2401.

Dale, A., Moore, P. P., Mcnicol, R. J., Sjulin, T. M., & Burmistrov, L. A. (1993). Genetic diversity of red raspberry varieties throughout the-world. *Journal of the American Society for Horticultural Science, 118*, 119–129.

Daskalova, E., Delchev, S., Topolov, M., Dimitrova, S., Uzunova, Y., Valcheva-Kuzmanova, S., Kratchanova, M., Vladimirova-Kitova, L., & Denev, P. (2019). Aronia melanocarpa (Michx.) Elliot fruit juice reveals neuroprotective effect and improves cognitive and locomotor functions of aged rats. *Food and Chemical Toxicology, 132*, 110674.

De Pascual-Teresa, S., Moreno, D. A., & Garcia-Viguera, C. (2010). Flavanols and anthocyanins in cardiovascular health: A review of current evidence. *International Journal of Molecular Sciences, 11*, 1679–1703.

Del Rio, D., Borges, G., & Crozier, A. (2010). Berry flavonoids and phenolics: Bioavailability and evidence of protective effects. *The British Journal of Nutrition, 104*(Suppl 3), S67–S90.

Devareddy, L., Hooshmand, S., Collins, J. K., Lucas, E. A., Chai, S. C., & Arjmandi, B. H. (2008). Blueberry prevents bone loss in ovariectomized rat model of postmenopausal osteoporosis. *The Journal of Nutritional Biochemistry, 19*, 694–699.

FDA. (2019). *Qualified health claims* [Online]. Food and Drug Administation. Available: https://www.fda.gov/food/food-labeling-nutrition/qualified-health-claims. Accessed January 2021.

FDA. (2020). *FDA announces qualified health claim for certain Cranberry products and urinary tract infections* [Online]. Food and Drug Administration. Available: https://www.fda.gov/food/cfsan-constituent-updates/fda-announces-qualified-health-claim-certain-cranberry-products-and-urinary-tract-infections. Accessed January 2021.

Ferlemi, A.-V., & Lamari, F. N. (2016). Berry leaves: An alternative source of bioactive natural products of nutritional and medicinal value. *Antioxidants, 5*, 17.

Fernandez, G. E., Garcia, E., & Lockwood, D. (2016). *Southeast regional Caneberry production guide*. NC Cooperative Extension Service.

Gao, N., Wang, Y., Jiao, X., Chou, S., Li, E., & Li, B. (2018). Preparative purification of polyphenols from Aronia melanocarpa (Chokeberry) with cellular antioxidant and antiproliferative activity. *Molecules, 23*, 139.

Hazen, R. A., Perkins, L. B., Bushway, R. J., & Bushway, A. A. (2004). Evaluation of water washes for the removal of organophosphorus pesticides from Maine wild blueberries. *Advances in Experimental Medicine and Biology, 542*, 309–315.

Hein, S., Whyte, A. R., Wood, E., Rodriguez-Mateos, A., & Williams, C. M. (2019). Systematic review of the effects of Blueberry on cognitive performance as we age. *The Journals of Gerontology. Series A, Biological Sciences and Medical Sciences, 74*, 984–995.

Hummer, K. E., & Barney, D. L. (2002). Currants. *Hort Technology, 12*, 377–387.

Johnson, S. A., Litwin, N. S., & Seals, D. R. (2019). Age-related vascular dysfunction: What registered dietitian nutritionists need to know. *Journal of the Academy of Nutrition and Dietetics, 119*, 1790–1796.

Kalt, W., Cassidy, A., Howard, L. R., Krikorian, R., Stull, A. J., Tremblay, F., & Zamora-Ros, R. (2020). Recent research on the health benefits of Blueberries and their anthocyanins. *Advances in Nutrition, 11*, 224–236.

Kim, H., Seo, K. H., & Yokoyama, W. (2020). Chemistry of pterostilbene and its metabolic effects. *Journal of Agricultural and Food Chemistry, 68*, 12836–12841.

King, E. S., & Bolling, B. W. (2020). Composition, polyphenol bioavailability, and health benefits of aronia berry: A review. *Journal of Food Bioactives, 11*.

Kokotkiewicz, A., Jaremicz, Z., & Luczkiewicz, M. (2010). Aronia plants: A review of traditional use, biological activities, and perspectives for modern medicine. *Journal of Medicinal Food, 13*, 255–269.

Kristo, A. S., Klimis-Zacas, D., & Sikalidis, A. K. (2016). *Protective role of dietary berries in cancer* (p. 5).

Kumar, N., & Goel, N. (2019). Phenolic acids: natural versatile molecules with promising therapeutic applications. *Biotechnology Reports (Amsterdam, Netherlands), 24*, e00370.

Lavefve, L., Howard, L. R., & Carbonero, F. (2020). Berry polyphenols metabolism and impact on human gut microbiota and health. *Food & Function, 11*, 45–65.

Lee, H. Y., Weon, J. B., Jung, Y. S., Kim, N. Y., Kim, M. K., & Ma, C. J. (2016). Cognitive-enhancing effect of Aronia melanocarpa extract against memory impairment induced by scopolamine in mice. *Evidence-based Complementary and Alternative Medicine, 2016*, 6145926.

Li, T., Wu, S.-M., Xu, Z.-Y., & Ou-Yang, S. (2014). Rabbiteye blueberry prevents osteoporosis in ovariectomized rats. *Journal of Orthopaedic Surgery and Research, 9*, 1–7.

Liu, Y., You, Y., Lu, J., Chen, X., & Yang, Z. (2020). Recent advances in synthesis, bioactivity, and pharmacokinetics of pterostilbene, an important analog of resveratrol. *Molecules, 25*.

Mainland, C. M. M. (2012). Frederick V. Coville and the history of North American highbush blueberry culture. *International Journal of Fruit Science, 12*, 4–13.

Manach, C., Scalbert, A., Morand, C., Remesy, C., & Jimenez, L. (2004). Polyphenols: food sources and bioavailability. *The American Journal of Clinical Nutrition, 79*, 727–747.

Mattioli, R., Francioso, A., Mosca, L., & Silva, P. (2020). Anthocyanins: A comprehensive review of their chemical properties and health effects on cardiovascular and neurodegenerative diseases. *Molecules, 25*.

Nauseda, E. (2020). Berry growers commit to 100% recycle-ready packaging. *Business Wire*.

Nestle, M. (2018). Superfoods are a marketing ploy. *The Atlantic*.

Paredes-López, O., Cervantes-Ceja, M. L., Vigna-Pérez, M., & Hernández-Pérez, T. (2010). Berries: Improving human health and healthy aging, and promoting quality life—A review. *Plant Foods for Human Nutrition, 65*, 299–308.

Piazza, S., Fumagalli, M., Khalilpour, S., Martinelli, G., Magnavacca, A., Dell'agli, M., & Sangiovanni, E. (2020). A review of the potential benefits of plants producing berries in skin disorders. *Antioxidants (Basel), 9*.

Robinson, J. A., Bierwirth, J. E., Greenspan, P., & Pegg, R. B. (2020). Blackberry polyphenols: Review of composition, quantity, and health impacts from in vitro and in vivo studies. *Journal of Food Bioactives, 9*.

Rodriguez-Mateos, A., Heiss, C., Borges, G., & Crozier, A. (2014). Berry (poly)phenols and cardiovascular health. *Journal of Agricultural and Food Chemistry, 62*, 3842–3851.

Sakaki, J., Melough, M., Lee, S. G., Kalinowski, J., Koo, S. I., Lee, S. K., & Chun, O. K. (2018). Blackcurrant supplementation improves trabecular bone mass in young but not aged mice. *Nutrients, 10*.

Shahin, L., Phaal, S. S., Vaidya, B. N., Brown, J. E., & Joshee, N. (2019). Aronia (Chokeberry): An underutilized, highly nutraceutical plant. *Journal of Medicinally Active Plants, 8*, 46–63.

Sidor, A., & Gramza-Michałowska, A. (2015). Advanced research on the antioxidant and health benefit of elderberry (Sambucus nigra) in food – A review. *Journal of Functional Foods, 18*, 941–958.

Singh, S., Virmani, T. & Kohli, K. (n.d.). Phytochemicals and medicinal uses of red raspberry: A review.

Speer, H., D'cunha, N. M., Alexopoulos, N. I., Mckune, A. J., & Naumovski, N. (2020). Anthocyanins and human health—A focus on oxidative stress, inflammation and disease. *Antioxidants, 9*, 366.

Strik, B. C. (2007). Berry crops: Worldwide area and production systems. *Berry Fruit Value Added Products for Health Promotion, 1*, 3–49.

Tasnim, R., Calderwood, L., Annis, S., Drummond, F., & Zhang, Y. (2020). The future of wild blueberries: Testing warming impacts using open-top chambers. *Spire*.

Umass-Extension. (2012). *Currants* [Online]. UMass Extension Center for Agriculture. Available: https://ag.umass.edu/sites/ag.umass.edu/files/fact-sheets/pdf/currants.pdf. Accessed January 2021.

Verma, R., Gangrade, T., Punasiya, R., & Ghulaxe, C. (2014). Rubus fruticosus (blackberry) use as an herbal medicine. *Pharmacognosy Reviews, 8*, 101–104.

Villata, M., & Council, U. H. B. (2012). Trends in world blueberry production. *Amer Fruit Growers, 132*, 30.

Vujanović, M., Majkić, T., Zengin, G., Beara, I., Tomović, V., Šojić, B., Đurović, S., & Radojković, M. (2020). Elderberry (Sambucus nigra L.) juice as a novel functional product rich in health-promoting compounds. *RSC Advances, 10*, 44805–44814.

Wood, E., Hein, S., Heiss, C., Williams, C., & Rodriguez-Mateos, A. (2019). Blueberries and cardiovascular disease prevention. *Food & Function, 10*, 7621–7633.

Zhang, J., Lazarenko, O. P., Blackburn, M. L., Shankar, K., Badger, T. M., Ronis, M. J., & Chen, J.-R. (2011). Feeding blueberry diets in early life prevent senescence of osteoblasts and bone loss in ovariectomized adult female rats. *PLoS One, 6*, e24486.

Zhang, J., Lazarenko, O. P., Kang, J., Blackburn, M. L., Ronis, M. J., Badger, T. M., & Chen, J.-R. (2013). Feeding blueberry diets to young rats dose-dependently inhibits bone resorption through suppression of RANKL in stromal cells. *PLoS One, 8*, e70438.

Zhao, Y. (2007). *Berry fruit: value-added products for health promotion*. CRC Press.

Zheng, X., Mun, S., Lee, S. G., Vance, T. M., Hubert, P., Koo, S. I., Lee, S. K., & Chun, O. K. (2016). Anthocyanin-rich Blackcurrant extract attenuates ovariectomy-induced bone loss in mice. *Journal of Medicinal Food, 19*, 390–397.

Chapter 4
Chocolate

Caitlin Clark

4.1 Cultural History

Archaeological evidence shows that the consumption of chocolate by humans has occurred for at least 5000 years, although it was almost certainly domesticated earlier and had already been in use for some time (Zarrillo et al., 2018, p. 1879). Recent findings show that cacao probably did not originate in Mexico as once presumed, but rather in the South American Amazon river basin. A single strain of cacao was brought north to Mesoamerica. This strain was cultivated first by the Olmecs and later the Maya, while older varieties remained in use in the Amazon (Zhang & Motilal, 2016, p. 8).

Chocolate began its slow transition into its modern form when Spanish conquistadores brought it back to Spain as a novelty beverage. Many of the early conquistadores, including Christopher Columbus, are rumored to have consumed cacao-based drinks with honey to reduce its bitterness. This tendency persisted when, in 1520, the conquistador Hernandos Cortés first introduced the beverage to Spain. Because of its rarity and high price, it was recognized as a status symbol and quickly spread amongst the upper classes. Only in the seventeenth century did chocolate reach the common classes and the rest of Europe (Afoakwa, 2016, p. 3).

Until the mid-nineteenth century, chocolate was still principally consumed as a beverage, although its popularity continued to expand (Afoakwa, 2016, p. 3). In 1847, Joseph Fry added additional sugar and cocoa butter to ground cacao beans to form the first edible solid chocolate bar, and the popularity of the confection soared further (Ozturk & Young, 2017, p. 433).

C. Clark (✉)
Colorado State University, Fort Collins, CO, USA
e-mail: Caitlin.Clark@colostate.edu

© The Author(s), under exclusive license to Springer Nature Switzerland AG 2022
J. P. Miller, C. Van Buiten (eds.), *Superfoods*, Food and Health,
https://doi.org/10.1007/978-3-030-93240-4_4

The innovation of milk chocolate by Daniel Peters in 1876 (Afoakwa, 2016, p. 3) and, shortly thereafter, the invention of the conche machine by Rudolph Lindt solidified chocolate's place as a global luxury (Beckett, 2009, p. 12). Milk powder, invented ten years earlier by Henri Nestlé, softened and smoothed the chocolate, completing its journey to the product we recognize today (Afoakwa, 2016, p. 3).

4.2   Current Research on Chocolate and Human Health

Over the years, chocolate has been used as everything from food, to ritual beverage, to medicine. Recently, chocolate has increasingly benefited from the halo of health associated with some of its constituent compounds, marking dark chocolate as a so-called "superfood". Indeed, the description applies only to dark chocolate. The health-associated compounds are sequestered in the cocoa solids; milk chocolate is comparatively low in cocoa solids (and high in unhealthy sugar and milk fats), while white chocolate contains no cocoa solids at all and classifies as chocolate only because it includes cocoa butter.

Chocolate is a complex food, with numerous compounds interacting to affect its nutritional and sensory qualities such as aroma and texture. Many of the individual components in chocolate have proven health effects or have been strongly correlated to positive outcomes when ingested. However, it is less obvious whether these components have the same effects when consumed as part of a chocolate matrix. More work needs to be done to link chocolate to health with the same confidence we apply to its individual constituent compounds.

The components in dark chocolate most strongly linked with health and well-being are two classes of compounds that are frequently associated with positive health outcomes: polyphenols (valued for antioxidant activity) and methylxanthines (recognized as stimulants). While these compounds may have some desirable health effects, it is important to understand them in context and also to describe how they affect the sensory aspects of finished chocolate.

4.2.1   Polyphenols

Polyphenols are the class of molecules perhaps most strongly associated, in the public consciousness, with the health benefits of chocolate. Compared to most foods, cacao hosts a rich abundance of these compounds: up to 10% of the dry weight of the cacao bean (Montagna et al., 2019, p. 4). This class of molecules has a number of healthful effects. They may reduce bodily markers of oxidative stress and protect against diabetes (Watson et al., 2013, pp. 327–354), and they have also been shown to help mobilize free fatty acids, the major fat fuel in the body, after exertion (Zugravu & Otelea, 2019, p. 1390). Polyphenols are likely to scavenge free radicals, which are unstable oxygen atoms that can damage cells or lead to illness and premature aging. Polyphenols are also able to chelate metals and trace elements, although the mechanisms of this have not been fully studied or described (Watson et al., 2013, p. 180). Some studies tout their effectiveness against cardiovascular disease (Watson et al., 2013, p. 192; Veronese et al., 2019, p. 1102). Two specific polyphenols, catechin and epicatechin, can cross the blood-brain barrier, and have been associated with improved vision, cognition, and neuroprotection (Zugravu & Otelea, 2019, p. 1391).

Chocolate is an excellent vehicle for polyphenol consumption, because while native cacao polyphenols have relatively low bioavailability (Rusconi & Conti, 2010, pp. 8–9), the simultaneous intake of sugar enhances polyphenol bioavailability and absorption in humans (Zugravu & Otelea, 2019, p. 1389).

While polyphenols generally have a positive association with health (except at extremely high doses), their contribution to chocolate sensory properties tends to be negative. High levels of any type of polyphenol can result in high perceived astringency and bitterness (Rusconi & Conti, 2010, p. 8; Caligiani et al., 2015, p. 186). For this reason, certain processing steps are carried out to reduce polyphenol content during chocolate-making. Raw cacao beans are extremely high in polyphenols; however, the processing of cacao into chocolate includes many steps (including fermentation, drying, conching, and the alkalization process known as dutching) which drastically reduce these antioxidant compounds, causing a decrease in their concentration. In addition, because cacao genetics, harvesting, and fermentation practices are different in every region, the amount of antioxidant polyphenol compounds in chocolate is hugely variable and sometimes as low as 0% (Rusconi & Conti, 2010, p. 7; Barišić et al., 2019, pp. 6–7). It is very difficult to guarantee the polyphenol content of a given piece of chocolate, despite its common recommendation by nutritionists as a polyphenol-rich "superfood".

Although more research is needed, an intriguing 2013 study suggested that a diet incorporating more than 650 milligrams of polyphenols per day was tied to a 30% reduction in mortality among adults (Zamora-Ros et al., 2013, pp. 1445–1450). Rusconi and Conti (2010, p. 6) show that dark chocolate polyphenol concentration averages approximately 1 g/100 g, or 0.5 g (500 mg) per 50 g bar. Even if we assume that all of those polyphenols are bioavailable (which is unlikely), this means that eating an entire chocolate bar per day still does not achieve the desired polyphenol consumption rate of 650 mg/day recommended by Zamora-Ros et al. (2013, pp. 1445–1450). However, dark chocolate has been used as part of a high-polyphenol diet in other nutrition regimens, in combination with polyphenol-rich fruits and vegetables (Kontogianni et al., 2020, pp. 1–16).

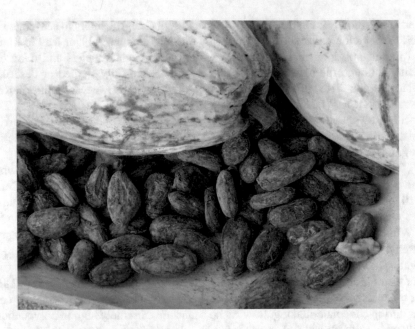

Photo by Joel (username) on Flickr (CC by 2.0)

4.2.2 Methylxanthines

Another class of bioactive compounds often associated with chocolate are the methylxanthine alkaloids: caffeine and theobromine. Dark chocolate contains about 19 mg of caffeine and 125–190 mg of theobromine per 25 g of chocolate; this is about half a typical chocolate bar (Aprotosoaie et al., 2016, p. 78). Both compounds have been found to stimulate nervous function, although they do so differently. While caffeine acts principally on the central nervous system, theobromine is a smooth muscle stimulant. Drinking chocolate beverages can improve cognitive function and reduce mental fatigue, and consumption of methylxanthines has been shown to reduce stress-related mediators (like cortisol) in highly anxious people (Zugravu & Otelea, 2019, p. 1391). Some chocolate consumers may also be relieved to find out that small doses of methylxanthines, such as those in chocolate, increase basal metabolic rates (Watson et al., 2013, p. 518). On the other hand, several compounds in chocolate, including methylxanthines, have also been recorded as migraine triggers (Zugravu & Otelea, 2019, p. 1392).

Both of the methylxanthines (caffeine and theobromine) in chocolate contribute to some of the bitterness in taste, but they are both also strongly associated with chocolate's "addictive" properties possibly due to their gentle psychoactive mechanism (Watson et al., 2013, p. 423). Amounts of methylxanthine equivalent to those in a 50 g chocolate bar strongly contribute to hedonic preference (liking) for chocolate. These compounds are thought to be linked to the acquired taste for chocolate that is not entirely explained only by its high content of sugar and fat (Smit & Blackburn, 2005, p. 104–105).

4.3 Related Topics

4.3.1 Botany

The cacao tree used in modern chocolate confectionary production is *Theobroma cacao*, and it is just one of the 22 species in the *Theobroma* family (Pérez-Mora et al., 2018, p. 496). *T. cacao* is the only *Theobroma* species widely cultivated, although several others are commonly used in parts of Central America to make chocolate or chocolate-like products, especially beverages such as Oaxacan tejate, which utilizes the seeds of *Theobroma bicolor* for their excellent foaming properties (Soleri & Cleveland, 2007, p. 113).

Cacao was once thought to fall into two main genetic groups, "Criollo" (meaning "first-grown" in Spanish) and "Forastero" (or "foreigner" in Spanish). A third group, "Trinitario", was thought to have resulted from an open-pollination hybridization of Criollo and Forastero on the island of Trinidad, for which it was named. However, seminal work by Motamayor et al. (2008, p. 2) analyzed numerous samples and found ten distinct genetic clusters: Amelonado, Contamana, Criollo, Curacay, Guiana, Iquiitos, Marañon, Nacional, Nanay, and Purús. Since then, unique genetic clusters have also been identified in Colombia (Osorio-Guarín et al., 2017, p. 11) Peru, and Bolivia (Zhang et al., 2010, p. 251).

Three cacao varieties, Criollo, Marañon, and Nacional, are known as "fine flavor" varieties because they produce highly desirable, pale, aromatic cacao beans that are low in bitterness and astringency. These varieties make up only 5% of global cacao production (Cadby & Araki, 2020, p. 2). World cacao production is largely made up of "bulk" cacao, including clone CCN-51. This hybrid was first developed in 1960s Ecuador and is known as CCN-51 for Colleción Castro Naranjal number 51 (Scharf et al., 2020, p. 1). Generally considered to have inferior organoleptic qualities, this cultivar is used only as "bulk cacao" and is preferred by the industrial producers rather than craft chocolate-makers (Jimenez et al., 2018, p. 2824).

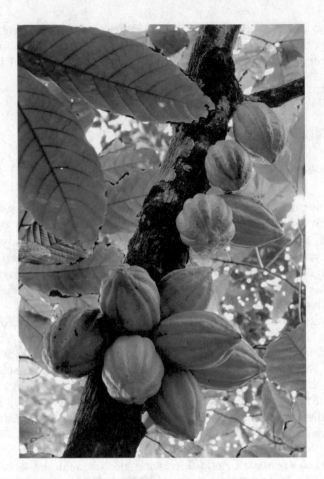

Photo by Luisovalles (username) via Wikimedia Commons (CC BY 3.0)

4.3.2   Fermentation

Many people remain unaware that cacao is a fermented food, sharing the distinction with such familiar favorites as cheese, soy sauce, and kombucha. In fact, the fermentation process converts the astringent, bitter seeds of the cacao tree into cacao beans—the raw material used to make chocolate. Without the fermentation step, cacao would taste shallow, empty, and decidedly unlike chocolate. (Afoakwa et al., 2008, p. 840).

Fermentation improves flavor by decomposing some of the bitter methylxanthine alkaloids and lowers astringency by breaking down polyphenols, levels of which can drop by as much as 70% in the fermentation step alone (Cornejo et al., 2018, p. 6). Fermentative breakdown of seed proteins facilitates Maillard reactions during roasting to form the nutty, roasted, compounds that give chocolate its characteristic flavor and aroma (Voigt et al., 1994, p. 204).

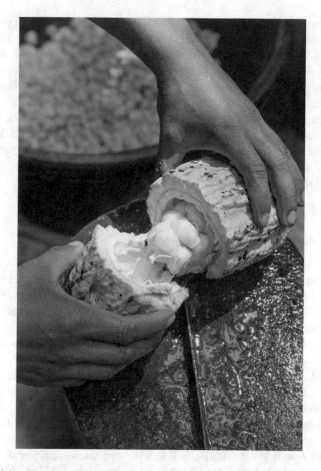

Photo by Rodrigo Flores on Unsplash

4.4 Social Issues

4.4.1 Cacao Farmers

Cacao farmers are among the poorest and lowest paid of all agriculture workers. Up to 90% of the world's seven million cacao farms are considered smallholders, maintaining family farms of less than 4 hectares, and frequently less than 2 hectares (Mortimer et al., 2018, p. 1640). Many have no official land titles, and the situation is even more tenuous for female farmers, who rarely retain legal control of their own farms. Tenure of a farm can be disrupted by civil war, unpredictable weather and climate conditions, or a shift in labor dynamics (Fountain & Hütz-Adams, 2018). Farmers are also susceptible to market changes that can leave them suddenly jobless or taking desperate measures to stay afloat. Especially in West African countries, whose economies depend substantially on sales of cacao and which are unable to easily recover from global downturns in demand, farmers experience loss of income without social protections (Duguma et al., 2001, p. 178). Often, farmers respond with an attempt to increase output, resulting in legal or illegal clearing of already threatened forests and the use of trafficked child labor to meet stretched production demands (Duguma et al., 2001, p. 178; Fountain & Hütz-Adams, 2018, pp. 16–18). In fact, the black market of child slavery has plagued the cacao sector for decades, despite repeated and unsubstantiated claims by multinational corporations and governments of cacao-producing countries that a solution is just over the horizon (Fountain & Hütz-Adams, 2018, pp. 16–18).

4.4.2   Environment and Agriculture

The *Theobroma cacao* tree is endemic to Central America but has now spread throughout the Americas, Western Africa, and parts of Asia and Indonesia. Its growing region extends 20° North and South of the equator, where temperatures average between 18° to 32 °C [64° to 90 °F] (Aprotosoaie et al., 2016, p. 73). Its yield is more affected by changes in rainfall than is the yield of many other species; it is not drought-tolerant and can endure dry spells of up to 3 months only.

Worldwide, about 70% of cacao is farmed under some type of shade or agroforestry system, because it is well-adapted to these conditions, being endemic to the Amazon rainforest (Mortimer et al., 2018, p. 1640; Arevalo-Gardini et al., 2019, p. 1). Since Beer et al. (1998, p. 146) reported that a shade cover of 40–70% provided ideal conditions, this has been the industry standard for cacao production. When such systems are put into practice, evidence shows that agroforestry techniques increase yields long-term (Rosenberg & Marcotte, 2005, p. 124). This has the added benefit of optimizing soil nutrients, slowing erosion, and the introduction of nitrogen-fixing species to the environment (Mortimer et al., 2018, p. 1645).

Moreover, agroforestry systems bring indirect benefits. Shade species may provide fruit, sap, or timber to supplement the income from cacao (Beer et al., 1998, p. 151). Farmers favor species such as citrus or mahogany that provide additional food and supplies for the homestead or can be sold for profit. Shade species also create leaf litter that contributes to nutrient cycling as well as improved water uptake for cacao trees due to vertical root segregation. Tertiary benefits include higher wildlife biodiversity, greater pollinator presence, and some advantages to pest control, although pests respond differently to forest environments and it is likely that further pest control measures should be taken (Mortimer et al., 2018, p. 1648).

The importance of agroforestry and shade management is proportional to the increasing heat and decreasing humidity of the growing region (Beer et al., 1998, pp. 146–147). This, along with social and historical factors, make the problem particularly relevant in Western and Central Africa. Cacao is an important cash crop that is essential to the economies of Ghana, Cote d'Ivoire, Nigeria, and Cameroon, among others. In these regions, yield per hectare averages lower than in the world's other cacao growing regions, weighing in at only 300–400 kg/ha as opposed to 500 kg/ha in Asia and up to 600 kg/ha in Central America (Cocoa Market Update, 2014, p. 2).

As a direct result of these adversities, farmers with limited access to diverse income opportunities are forced to continually forsake existing crops and expand the territory of their farmsteads to areas where soil nutrients are less depleted. Farmers regularly abandon trees that have withered due to lack of shade management and start new crops, applying a form of slash-and-burn agriculture that has diminished West Africa's original forests by 90% (Fountain & Hütz-Adams, 2018, p. 18). With so little potentially farmable land remaining, this cycle is quickly consuming the remaining forest area of Western Africa and turning cacao farming into a blood sport.

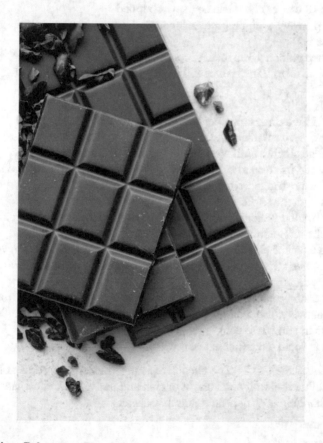

Photo by Tetiana Bykovets on Unsplash

4.5   Recipes

Simple Truffle   Truffles are simply a ball of sweetened chocolate ganache with an edible coating. This could be another layer of chocolate or coconut or—for a traditional spin—cocoa powder. Texture is key to a truffle's success; you will note that the ingredients call for "golden syrup, honey or another form of invert syrup". An invert syrup is a sugar syrup in which the disaccharide sucrose (table sugar) has been converted to its constituent monosaccharide molecules of glucose and fructose. This causes it to taste sweeter but more importantly, it prevents re-crystallization of the dissolved sugar, which keeps the chocolate ganache smooth and silky.

Servings: About 30
Ingredients:

- 0.5 lb. (8 oz.) of chocolate coarsely chopped
- 2 Tbsp heavy whipping cream (coconut cream works well as a non-dairy alternative)
- 1.5 Tbsp golden syrup, honey, corn syrup, or other invert sugar
- Optional: up to 1 Tbsp butter will improve the texture and shine of your ganache

Instructions:

1. Mix all ingredients together in a microwave-safe bowl.
2. Microwave until melted, stirring at 30-second intervals.
3. Continue stirring until the mixture has begun to thicken slightly.
4. Allow the mixture to cool at room temperature or in the refrigerator (if you choose the fridge, avoid condensation by placing a layer of plastic wrap directly on the surface).
5. Use a melon baller or two spoons to scoop pieces of cooled and hardened ganache into mounds about 1 Tablespoon in size.
6. Using clean or gloved hands, roll each mound into a ball. Don't worry if they are not perfectly round! It is both attractive and traditional for truffles to be slightly misshapen.
7. Roll each ganache ball in cocoa powder, coconut, or crushed nuts. Alternatively, use a dipping tool or fork to dip each ball in tempered chocolate, then allow it to cool.
8. Store at room temperature at eat within 3–4 days for best quality.

Flourless Chocolate Cake   The chocolate really shines here, so use one that you love, whether it is fruity and bright or rich and nutty. Dark chocolate works best but try changing it up depending on the season.

Servings: 6–8
Ingredients:

- 8 eggs, kept cold
- 1 lb. (16 oz.) of chocolate (preferably dark), coarsely chopped

- 16 Tbsp unsalted butter, cut into 12–16 pieces
- Optional: powdered sugar, orange slices, or berries for topping

Instructions:

1. Heat your oven to 325 °F and place your oven rack as close to the middle of the oven as possible. Line the base of an 8-inch springform pan with parchment paper. Grease the pan very well, all along the sides and the lined bottom. Then, wrap the outside of the springform pan in several layers of aluminum foil and set it in a larger pan (such as a roasting pan). This will form your bain-marie. Boil some water while you prepare the batter.
2. Beat the eggs until they have doubled in volume (about 5 minutes). This is best done with the whisk attachment of a stand mixer. This step is crucial to the texture of the cake.
3. While the eggs are beating, melt the butter and chocolate together over a double boiler or in a microwave, stirring at 30-second intervals.
4. Fold 1/3 of the eggs into the melted chocolate mixture and stir until smooth and you see very few streaks of eggs. Repeat with another 1/3 of the egg mixture (half of the remaining mixture), then finally fold in the last of the egg mixture, folding gently until the batter is completely homogenous.
5. Pour the batter into the springform pan, scraping with a silicone or rubber spatula. Then, place the springform pan into the larger pan, and pour in enough boiling water that it reaches halfway up the sides of the springform pan. Do this carefully! Water should not splash into the batter mixture.
6. Bake for 22–26 minutes until the edges of the cake are just beginning to set and the cake has risen. You should see a crust barely forming on the surface. When the cake is done, an instant-read thermometer inserted in the center will show 140 °F. At this point, carefully withdraw the cake from the bain-marie and allow it to cool completely before removing the springform pan.
7. Top the cooled cake with powdered sugar, whipped cream, berries, or coulis as desired.

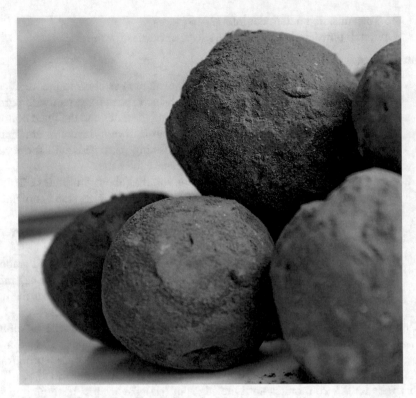

Photo by Hannah Dodwell on Unsplash

References

Afoakwa, E. O. (2016). *Chocolate science and technology* (2nd ed.). Accra.

Afoakwa, E. O., Paterson, A., Fowler, M., & Ryan, A. (2008). Flavor formation and character in cocoa and chocolate: A critical review. *Critical Reviews in Food Science and Nutrition, 48*(9), 840–857. https://doi.org/10.1080/10408390701719272

Aprotosoaie, A. C., Luca, S. V., & Miron, A. (2016). Flavor chemistry of cocoa and cocoa products – An overview. *Comprehensive Reviews in Food Science and Food Safety, 15*(1), 73–91. https://doi.org/10.1111/1541-4337.12180

Arevalo-Gardini, E., Meinhardt, L. W., Zuñiga, L. C., Arévalo-Gardni, J., Motilal, L., & Zhang, D. (2019). Genetic identity and origin of "Piura Porcelana"— A fine-flavored traditional variety of cacao (Theobroma cacao) from the Peruvian Amazon. *Tree Genetics & Genomes, 15*(1). https://doi.org/10.1007/s11295-019-1316-y

Barišić, V., Kopjar, M., Jozinović, A., Flanjak, I., Ačkar, Đ., Miličević, B., … Babić, J. (2019). The chemistry behind chocolate production. *Molecules, 24*(17). https://doi.org/10.3390/molecules24173163

Beckett, S. T. (2009). Industrial chocolate manufacture and use. In S. T. Beckett (Ed.), *Industrial chocolate manufacture and use* (4th ed.). Blackwell Publishing Ltd.

Beer, J., Kass, D. C., Muschler, R., & Somarriba, E. J. (1998). Shade management in coffee and Cacao plantations. *Agroforestry Systems, 38*, 139–164.

Cadby, J., & Araki, T. (2020). *Towards ethical chocolate: Multicriterial identifiers, pricing structures, and the role of the specialty cacao industry in sustainable development. SN Business & Economics.* Springer International Publishing. https://doi.org/10.1007/s43546-021-00051-y

Caligiani, A., Marseglia, A., & Palla, G. (2015). Cocoa: production, chemistry, and use. In *Encyclopedia of food and health* (pp. 185–190). https://doi.org/10.1016/B978-0-12-384947-2.00177-X

Cocoa Market Update. (2014). Retrieved from www.WorldCocoa.org

Cornejo, O. E., Yee, M. C., Dominguez, V., Andrews, M., Sockell, A., Strandberg, E., … Motamayor, J. C. (2018). Population genomic analyses of the chocolate tree, Theobroma cacao L., provide insights into its domestication process. *Communications Biology, 1*(1), 1–12. https://doi.org/10.1038/s42003-018-0168-6

Duguma, B., Gockowski, J., & Bakala, J. (2001). Smallholder cacao (Theobroma cacao Linn.) cultivation in agroforestry systems of West and Central Africa: Challenges and opportunities. *Agroforestry Systems, 51*(3), 177–188. https://doi.org/10.1023/A:1010747224249

Fountain, A. C., & Hütz-Adams, F. (2018). *Cocoa Barometer 2018.* Retrieved from http://www.cocoabarometer.org/Cocoa_Barometer/Download_files/2018 Cocoa Barometer 180420.pdf

Jimenez, J. C., Amores, F. M., Solórzano, E. G., Rodríguez, G. A., La Mantia, A., Blasi, P., & Loor, R. G. (2018). Differentiation of Ecuadorian National and CCN-51 cocoa beans and their mixtures by computer vision. *Journal of the Science of Food and Agriculture, 98*(7), 2824–2829. https://doi.org/10.1002/jsfa.8790

Kontogianni, M. D., Vijayakumar, A., Rooney, C., Noad, R. L., Appleton, K. M., McCarthy, D., … Woodside, J. V. (2020). A high polyphenol diet improves psychological well-being: The polyphenol intervention trial (pphit). *Nutrients, 12*(8), 1–16. https://doi.org/10.3390/nu12082445

Montagna, M. T., Diella, G., Triggiano, F., Caponio, G. R., De Giglio, O., Caggiano, G., … Portincasa, P. (2019). Chocolate, "food of the gods": History, science, and human health. *International Journal of Environmental Research and Public Health, 16*(24). https://doi.org/10.3390/ijerph16244960

Mortimer, R., Saj, S., & David, C. (2018). Supporting and regulating ecosystem services in cacao agroforestry systems. *Agroforestry Systems, 92*(6), 1639–1657. https://doi.org/10.1007/s10457-017-0113-6

Motamayor, J. C., Lachenaud, P., da Silva e Mota, J., Loor, R., Kuhn, D. N., Brown, J. S., & Schnell, R. J. (2008). Geographic and genetic population differentiation of the Amazonian chocolate tree (Theobroma cacao L). *PLoS One, 3*(10), 1–8. https://doi.org/10.1371/journal.pone.0003311

Osorio-Guarín, J. A., Berdugo-Cely, J., Coronado, R. A., Zapata, Y. P., Quintero, C., Gallego-Sánchez, G., & Yockteng, R. (2017). Colombia a source of cacao genetic diversity as revealed by the population structure analysis of germplasm bank of Theobroma cacao l. *Frontiers in Plant Science, 8*(November), 1994. https://doi.org/10.3389/fpls.2017.01994

Ozturk, G., & Young, G. M. (2017, May 1). Food evolution: The impact of society and science on the fermentation of Cocoa beans. *Comprehensive reviews in food science and food safety.* John Wiley & Sons, Ltd (10.1111). https://doi.org/10.1111/1541-4337.12264

Pérez-Mora, W., Jorrin-Novo, J. V., & Melgarejo, L. M. (2018). Substantial equivalence analysis in fruits from three Theobroma species through chemical composition and protein profiling. *Food Chemistry, 240*, 496–504. https://doi.org/10.1016/j.foodchem.2017.07.128

Rosenberg, D. E., & Marcotte, T. P. (2005). Land-use system modeling and analysis of shaded cacao production in Belize. *Agroforestry Systems, 64*(2), 117–129. https://doi.org/10.1007/s10457-004-0535-9

Rusconi, M., & Conti, A. (2010, January 1). Theobroma cacao L., the food of the Gods: A scientific approach beyond myths and claims. *Pharmacological Research.* Academic Press. https://doi.org/10.1016/j.phrs.2009.08.008

Scharf, A., Lang, C., & Fischer, M. (2020). Genetic authentication: Differentiation of fine and bulk cocoa (Theobroma cacao L.) by a new CRISPR/Cas9-based in vitro method. *Food Control, 114*, 1–9. https://doi.org/10.1016/j.foodcont.2020.107219

Smit, H. J., & Blackburn, R. J. (2005). Reinforcing effects of caffeine and theobromine as found in chocolate. *Psychopharmacology, 181*(1), 101–106. https://doi.org/10.1007/s00213-005-2209-3

Soleri, D., & Cleveland, D. A. (2007). Tejate: Theobroma cacao and T. Bicolor in a traditional beverage from Oaxaca, Mexico. *Food and Foodways, 15*(1–2), 107–118. https://doi.org/10.1080/07409710701260131

Veronese, N., Demurtas, J., Celotto, S., Caruso, M. G., Maggi, S., Bolzetta, F., … Stubbs, B. (2019). Is chocolate consumption associated with health outcomes? An umbrella review of systematic reviews and meta-analyses. *Clinical Nutrition, 38*(3), 1101–1108. https://doi.org/10.1016/j.clnu.2018.05.019

Voigt, J., Heinrichs, H., Voigt, G., & Biehl, B. (1994). Cocoa-specific aroma precursors are generated by proteolytic digestion of the vicilin-like globulin of cocoa seeds. *Food Chemistry, 50*(2), 177–184. https://doi.org/10.1016/0308-8146(94)90117-1

Watson, R. R., Preedy, V. R., & Zibadi, S. (Eds.). (2013). Chocolate in health and nutrition. *Chocolate in Health and Nutrition.* https://doi.org/10.1007/978-1-61779-803-0_4

Zamora-Ros, R., Rabassa, M., Cherubini, A., Urpí-Sardà, M., Bandinelli, S., Ferrucci, L., & Andres-Lacueva, C. (2013). High concentrations of a urinary biomarker of polyphenol intake are associated with decreased mortality in older adults. *The Journal of Nutrition, 143*(9), 1445–1450. https://doi.org/10.3945/jn.113.177121

Zarrillo, S., Gaikwad, N., Lanaud, C., Powis, T., Viot, C., Lesur, I., … Valdez, F. (2018). The use and domestication of Theobroma cacao during the mid-Holocene in the upper Amazon. *Nature Ecology and Evolution, 2*(12), 1879–1888. https://doi.org/10.1038/s41559-018-0697-x

Zhang, D., & Motilal, L. (2016). Origin, dispersal, and current global distribution of cacao genetic diversity. In *Cacao diseases: a history of old enemies and new encounters* (pp. 3–31). Springer International Publishing. https://doi.org/10.1007/978-3-319-24789-2_1

Zhang, D., Gardini, E. A., Motilal, L. A., Baligar, V., Bailey, B., Zuñiga-Cernades, L., … Meinhardt, L. (2010). Dissecting genetic structure in farmer selections of Theobroma Cacao in the Peruvian Amazon: implications for on farm conservation and rehabilitation. *Tropical Plant Biology, 4*(2), 106–116. https://doi.org/10.1007/s12042-010-9064-z

Zugravu, C., & Otelea, M. R. (2019). Dark chocolate: To eat or not to eat? A review. *Journal of AOAC International, 102*(5), 1388–1396. https://doi.org/10.5740/jaoacint.19-0132

Chapter 5
Coffee

Walter F. Carroll

Coffee is a global beverage with a long, sometimes dark, history. Coffee "is grown commercially on four continents and consumed enthusiastically on all seven" (Morris 2018, p. 7), but most coffee consumption occurs in the developed countries of the world, the Global North, with the United States leading. People in the less developed world, the Global South, drink less coffee. Rather, they grow and produce the beverage based on the coffee bean, or cherry. That difference is crucial for understanding the history and current standing of coffee as a global beverage and commodity. Caffeine, which provides a lift and heightens concentration, helps to explain coffee's success since its discovery in East Africa around 850 CE.

5.1 Coffee: A Cultural History

Although no one knows for sure when, where, and how coffee was discovered, most agree it emerged in Ethiopia. Morris (2018) divides the history of coffee into five eras after its initial discovery. The first encompasses the onset of commercial production in Yemen and its spread throughout the Middle East and Northern Africa. That era was succeeded by the colonial period during which European countries forced their subjects to produce coffee. The repercussions of that era remain with us. In the third era, increasing coffee output in Brazil led to coffee emerging as an industrial product heavily consumed in North America. In the fourth era, Asia and Africa began to play significant roles in coffee production and trading. Finally, Morris suggests that a fifth incipient era may signal the development of high-end, specialty coffees with worldwide appeal.

W. F. Carroll (✉)
Bridgewater State University, Bridgewater, MA, USA
e-mail: wcarroll@bridgew.edu

© The Author(s), under exclusive license to Springer Nature Switzerland AG 2022
J. P. Miller, C. Van Buiten (eds.), *Superfoods*, Food and Health,
https://doi.org/10.1007/978-3-030-93240-4_5

Juma (1989, p. 41) fleshes out that overview, summarizing the early years of coffee including its discovery and spread:

> Coffee (*Coffea arabica*) originated in the highlands of Ethiopia and was first domesticated in the Arab world; from there it presumably reached India. The Dutch found the plant in India and planted it in Ceylon in 1659 and Java in 1696. A single coffee tree which reached the Amsterdam Botanical Garden in 1706 was later the basis of most of the coffee grown in South America. Seeds from the plant were first sent to Surinam in 1715, and coffee trees from Surinam were transferred to Brazil in 1727. Seeds from the same tree in Amsterdam went to the Jardin Royal in Paris and subsequently to Martinique in 1723.

Most agree with Juma that coffee originated in Ethiopia, but no one really knows how coffee was discovered. The most widely known and probably the most pleasing story revolves around a goat herder named Kaldi. Noticing that his goats had been very active and frisky as they clustered around and ate berries from a particular bush, he also tried the berries and discovered the jolt that caffeine has been delivering since then. Coffee, produced commercially in Yemen, spread throughout the Middle East, Northern Africa, and India, and became known as the "Wine of Islam," owing to the Islamic prohibition on alcohol consumption. Hattox (2014) notes its wide use in Yemen, usually tied to the Sufi order of Islam. Sufi mystics participated in ceremonies for long hours and well into the night, but they worked during the day. The caffeine in coffee helped they stay awake and alert.

When Europeans first encountered coffee in the Middle East, often in coffeehouses, many were repulsed by it. But in 1652, coffeehouse culture began to spread to London and Ellis (2011) notes in his cultural history of coffeehouses how a "simple commodity rewrote the experience of metropolitan life." As the appeal of coffee spread, European countries began producing the increasingly valuable plant in their colonies. Juma refers to two aspects of the role of colonialism in the rise of coffee as a global commodity. The obvious point is that European countries, starting with the Netherlands, forced those under their control to grow coffee, but there is also the sense that European control included bringing seeds and plants, specifically in this case, coffee plants, from various areas of the world back to Europe.

Under colonialism during the late seventeenth and the eighteenth centuries, Europeans used force, coercion, and, at times, slavery to force subject peoples to grow and produce coffee. This led to the globalizing of coffee while creating problems in the colonies in which it was grown, problems that remain today. For example, indigenous people were often forced to abandon agricultural production based on subsistence that they had used for centuries and that had enabled them to live in sustainable ways. Imposed coffee monocultures upended their lives, their existing means of food production, and their cultures. Where slavery was imposed, such as Brazil, many African slaves perished. Thus, "coffee became a major global commodity through a long and complicated historical process lasting centuries and entailing the gradual expansion of production and consumption, alongside new developments in international transportation, shipping, processing, and grading" (Fridell, 2014, p. 25).

North America and Europe became the core coffee consuming regions in the nineteenth century, succeeding the dominance of the "nearly three hundred years prior to that when the international coffee trade was dominated by Indian and Arab merchants linking growers in Ethiopia and Yemen with major markets in the Middle East and North Africa," (Fridell, 2014, p. 26). Shifting to Morris' fourth era, coffee became a global industrial product largely produced in tropical zones and primarily consumed in the temperate zones of the Global North.

During this period the largest producer of coffee was Brazil followed by other Latin American countries, such as Colombia. Brazil is still the world's largest producer of coffee beans, but Vietnam is now second, based on a shift to growing Robusta starting in the 1950s. That led to both Asia and Africa becoming coffee producers and exporters.

Morris suggests that the fifth era could see coffee as a product consumed globally. That process is ongoing with growing numbers of people outside of North America and Europe drinking coffee and many in those areas purchasing their own beans or enjoying their coffee in specialty shops.

5.2 The Current State of Nutritional Research on Coffee and Its Health Claims

Thousands of scientific studies of coffee's effects indicate that not only is it not harmful, but, when consumed in reasonable amounts, it confers positive health effects. Although scientific research continues and debates over coffee and caffeine recur, recent scientific reviews of research support the consensus about coffee drinking and caffeine consumption. Jane Brody, the *New York Times* Personal Health writer sums up that consensus in the print title of her article "Wake Up to the Good News about Coffee" (2021). The subhead of the online version of the article notes that "Drinking coffee has been linked to a reduced risk of all kinds of ailments, including Parkinson's disease, melatonin, prostate cancer, even suicide." One core issue in assessing the effects of coffee is the level of consumption, with 400 milligrams – four or five cups – generally considered the safe maximum daily consumption.

Brody notes that over the years there have been scares about the effects of coffee, including suggestions that it causes a myriad of conditions, including "heart disease, stroke, Type 2 diabetes, pancreatic cancer, anxiety disorder, nutrient deficiencies, gastric reflux disease, migraine, insomnia, and premature death" (2021). Reviews of the effects of coffee and caffeine include "Coffee, Caffeine, and Health Outcomes: An Umbrella Review," in the *Annual Review of Nutrition*," (Grosso et al., 2017) and "Coffee, Caffeine, and Health," in the *New England Journal of Medicine* (NEJM) (van Dam et al., 2020). Grosso et al. (2017) found coffee consumption associated with decreases in various types of cancer, cardiovascular disease and mortality, Parkinson's disease, and type 2 diabetes. The authors of the Umbrella review conclude that "coffee can be part of a healthful diet" (Grosso et al., 2017, p. 131). The journal *Nutrients* published a special issue examining "The

Impact of Caffeine and Coffee on Human Health" (Bamia & Cornelis, 2019). Nine reviews of literature and 10 original research articles in the issue explore the complexities of coffee's effects, but generally agree that in appropriate amounts it is safe.

Dr. Walter C. Willet, professor of nutrition and epidemiology at the Harvard T.H. Chan School of Public Health, notes the periodic scares about coffee "'have given the public a very distorted view'" (Brody, 2021). Based on the results of the research reviews and echoing Brody's comments he argues that "overall, despite various concerns that have cropped up over the years, coffee is remarkably safe and has a number of important potential benefits."

Further supporting the consensus, the Harvard T.H. Chan School of Public Health on its Nutrition Source webpage, suggests that "coffee is a healthy choice for most people" and that "consumption of 3 to 5 standard cups of coffee daily has been consistently associated with a reduced risk of several chronic diseases," (Harvard T.H. Chan, 2021). Edward Giovannucci, a professor of epidemiology and nutrition at the Chan school, as reported in a Consumer Reports article, also concluded that coffee seems to be healthy (Cook, 2019).

The research suggesting the safety and positive health outcomes of coffee and caffeine consumption does not mean that there are no possible problems with coffee consumption. One area of concern is the effects of coffee on pregnant women. The studies listed above did find increased risk of pregnancy loss, suggesting the importance of following the guidelines of the American College of Obstetricians and Gynecologists (ACOG) that drinking 200 milligrams of coffee (about 1–2 cups) a day, or 12 ounces, is safe during pregnancy (ACOG, 2020). Originally issued in 2010, the guidelines were affirmed in 2020.

In 2008, the *American Journal of Obstetrics and Gynecology* published an article suggesting that increasing caffeine consumption during pregnancy was associated with increased risks of miscarriages (Weng et al., 2008). A note in the *New York Times* drew additional attention to the article (Grady, 2008) which recommended that pregnant women avoid coffee. In addition to the ACOG declining to alter its guidelines, two obstetricians reacted with a letter on "Coffee Pregnancy," to the *New York Times* (Klatsky & Tran, 2008) noting "that findings like these generate more media coverage because of the interest and fear they generate, rather than the quality of the evidence." Dr. Carolyn Westhoff, professor of obstetrics, gynecology, and epidemiology at Columbia University Medical Center expressed reservations about the study "noting that miscarriage is difficult to study or explain" (Grady, 2008).

More recently an *MBJ Evidence-Based Medicine* article reviewed the evidence on pregnancy and coffee and caffeine consumption (James, 2020) and suggested that caffeine consumption was dangerous to pregnant women, leading to a greater likelihood of six negative outcomes: miscarriage, still birth, low birth weight, preterm birth, childhood acute leukemia, and of having an overweight child. The research review garnered attention, but again the ACOG did not concur. A key problem was that most of the studies reviewed were observational rather than experimental studies which makes it difficult to draw unequivocal conclusions. The ACOG recommendations seem judicious based on the evidence.

Looking at another aspect of coffee's effects on women, a study in the *European Journal of Cancer Prevention* (Abel et al., 2007) drew on a sample of over 93,000 women to investigate the relationship between daily coffee consumption and non-melanoma skin cancer among European American white women. Women who drank caffeinated coffee daily were 10.8% less likely to develop that cancer. Drinking noncaffeinated coffee did not confer the same advantage. A review examining research on the topic cautiously drew the conclusion that "coffee intake appears to exert a moderate protection against BCC [basal cell carcinoma] development, probably through the biological effects of caffeine" (Saverio et al., 2017), but urged caution because many of the studies were observational rather than randomized clinical trials and suggested that more such studies were warranted. That is obviously also the case for studying the impact of coffee on pregnant women.

5.3 Coffee: Botanical and Ecological Aspects

Coffee beans are cherries grown from plants called Coffea. The cherries, or beans, are originally green, but darken during roasting. Coffee is rich in various chemicals and substances that presumably give it the nutritional and health benefits that moderate consumption seems to produce. According to the Harvard T.H. Chan School (2021) "coffee is an intricate mixture of more than a thousand chemicals." Those include most prominently caffeine; but also, vitamin B12, known as riboflavin; magnesium; and a variety of plant chemicals. Van Dam et al. (2020) note that coffee contains "hundreds of other biologically active phytochemicals" which may contribute to its effects on health.

Caffeine is the best-known ingredient in coffee and seems to play a key role in conferring the health benefits of the beverage although other ingredients may play a role. In terms of caffeine's evolutionary success, Michael Pollan (2019), in his spoken word "Caffeine: How Caffeine Created the Modern World," notes that caffeine, "one of the most studied psychoactive compounds there is," succeeded by solving a problem that it created: caffeine withdrawal. Continuing caffeine consumption prevents that withdrawal and the unpleasant symptoms associated with it. It is, Pollan suggests, a botanical success story through evolution.

As part of that success story, for centuries people have experienced the sharpening of focus, the energy jolt, and the heightened concentration caffeine brings. The substance itself is a complicated bitter white power with the scientific name 1,3,7-trimethylpurine-2,6-dione. Caffeine enabled the survival of coffee plants by repulsing predators, but that protection may not last forever as predators continue to evolve to gain resistance, illustrating the Red Queen hypothesis that greater and greater efforts are necessary to maintain resistance (Dunn, 2017). That could lead to a story of failure through evolution.

While there are over 120 species of coffee bean, Arabica (*Coffea arabica*) is the most valued and considered to be the best tasting. Acknowledged as the hardest to grow, it accounts for about 60% of coffee production worldwide (Van der Vossen et al., 2015). The second most widely used is Robusta (*Coffea canephora*), now mostly used in cheaper coffee blends or in instant coffee. Robusta is frequently considered inferior to Arabica, but some experts believe Robusta is not inherently inferior and that when properly processed could be popular with consumers. Due to climate change, Robusta may become more important in the international coffee trade because it more tolerant of heat, erratic weather, and We T. Other varieties such as Liberian coffee (*Coffea liberica*) generally have even more caffeine and harsher taste.

Ecologist Rob Dunn (2017) argues that the monocultures can be dangerous to the cultivated plant itself. This happened with bananas where a monoculture led to the elimination of the Gros Michel species and the succession to Cavendish bananas. Dunn discusses the example of coffee in Sri Lanka, formerly known as Ceylon, an area where colonizers forced the production of coffee as a monoculture. The biological problems growing only one variant of a plan affected coffee by the eighteenth century. The British took Ceylon from the Dutch in 1797. Responding to increasing demand the British expanded coffee production and planted coffee in large monocultures, despite warnings from a British fungal biologist, Harry Marshal Ward. His argument then has relevance today in a world of waning biodiversity. With monocultures if a pest or pathogen affects one plant, such as coffee, it could kill all the plants and the predators keep evolving to pose greater threats.

Dunn notes that "coffee rust wiped out the coffee of Ceylon and, subsequently, much of the rest of the coffee of Asia and Africa. Coffee growers replanted with tea" (Dunn, 2017, p. 7). Even with the earlier examples of coffee and other plants illustrating the dangers of a lack of biodiversity, coffee remains at risk today. "Having learned nothing from Sri Lanka, we have once more planted varieties of coffee that are susceptible to coffee rust in large plantations, and the rust is back." That various plants, including coffee, are at risk today from "pests, pathogens, and climate change is not a fluke. Given our preferences, it was inevitable" (Dunn, 2017, p. 11).

Coffee now faces many threats, from, for example,

> the coffee berry borer, a beetle that burrows into the seeds of coffee – where it uses a fungus to detoxify the coffee's caffeine and then eats to its tiny, simple heart's content – many other insects, and a rust, the same rust that destroyed coffee in what is now Sri Lanka in the 1880s, where Arabica coffee was being grown. The rust appears to be nearly unstoppable (Dunn, 2017, pp. 98–99).

To combat earlier threats to Arabica growers switched to coffees that were resistant to rust, such as Liberian coffee, but the resistance was short-lived. Farmers also switched to Robusta, which was resistant but is less flavorful than Arabica. The rust is evolving and now attacking all coffees. Coffee is still doing well in Latin America, but the future there may also be uncertain.

5.4   Coffee and Social Issues

Fridell (2014, p. 5) notes that coffee is the classic global commodity. Produced as a universal good for sale on the market, "it links the daily routine of millions of consumers and producers living thousands of kilometers apart and experiencing vastly different lives." Those vastly different lives, the nature of coffee production and consumption, and the operations of the global coffee market generate social issues and problems for many. Coffee generates huge sums of money, "and yet, despite billions of dollars in profits made each year, the majority of the world's coffee families live in relative poverty. Who is the culprit for such vast inequality?" (Fridell, 2014, p. 5). Anthropologist Catherine M. Tucker summarizes the profound social issues associated with coffee cultivation, processing, and trade as "social inequality, biodiversity conservation, and environmental degradation" (Tucker, 2011, p. xii).

The demands of production for the global market make it difficult for cultivators who in the past might have at least partially engaged in subsistence production to feed themselves and their families. The fluctuations of coffee markets determine the fortunes of many of the cultivators. A glut of beans on global markets causes prices to drop, and those at the bottom of this economy suffer the most. If coffee producing countries flood the market with coffee beans, prices plummet and at times coffee must be discarded. This is often explained as regrettable, but just the way that markets work and it's not really anyone's fault and probably cannot be changed. This line of neoliberal reasoning emphasizes the importance of free trade and freely operating markets. Those taking this approach, whether trade economists, states, or coffee corporations, argue that calls for state intervention or regulation of coffee markets and the coffee industry are misguided, have not worked, and would not work.

Fridell (2014) notes that this ignores much recent research and discussion about the political economy of coffee. He argues that powerful states play an important role in the global coffee economy, as do private actors such as large coffee corporations. He discusses the International Coffee Agreement (ICA) that from 1962 to 1989 included most of the major coffee producing and consuming nations in efforts to minimize coffee price fluctuations. Despite its relative success in stabilizing prices, it was seen as too political and as interfering with free markets.

Fair Trade agreements seek to guarantee fair prices for coffee producers and have improved the situations for many, giving them greater income and opportunities for education, but, while these are well intentioned, questions arise about their overall effects. Only small percentages of coffee are certified as Fair Trade and those coffees cost consumers more limiting their appeal. Market-based solutions, however well intended, may not solve the inherent inequalities, lack of social justice, and environmental issues generated by the capitalist coffee economy.

Growing, processing, and trading coffee requires high levels of both natural and technological resources. These include petroleum, huge inputs of chemicals such as nitrogen, phosphorus, and potassium. The process of growing coffee itself has negative implications for the land and for sustainability (Tucker, 2011). Different methods of coffee cultivation entail different types of environmental costs, but overall, create major problems of environmental damage and sustainability.

These issues and others lead Tucker (2011, p. 118) to ask, "Given the relationships between coffee production and social tragedies, do you think it is possible to produce a commodity like coffee without economic problems or human suffering?" It is a difficult question to answer, but an important one to ponder. If it is not possible now, is there any way to make it possible?

5.5 Recipes

Making Coffee With so many specialty coffee cafes and roasters there is an incredible variety of coffee and coffee-related beverages available, but most of those drinks require trained baristas to produce. However, with the good coffee, the right equipment, and a few guidelines, one can make excellent coffee themselves. Here are some hints to aid in that.

There are many ways to make coffee. Expresso, coffee making machines, cold brew, and others have their adherents. Some types of coffee making are more appropriate for certain types of roasts or coffees than others. There are also capsule machines, but they make it difficult to make good coffee. Of all the approaches to making coffee, pour-over makes a bright, clean, flavorful coffee that appeals to many.

Pour over involves pouring hot water into a vessel through a filter. Chemex, Hario, and Bee House are among the most popular of the pour over methods and brands. Although each has idiosyncratic features and instructions, they are broadly similar and the keys to making a good pour over coffee are helpful for making any type of coffee. Various specialty coffee retailers provide guides to making pour over and other types of coffee on their websites. They also provide excellent beans.

Here are some pointers to making good coffee, pour over and others.

1. Buy whole beans that have been roasted as recently as possible.
2. Store the beans at room temperature and out of direct sunlight.
3. Grind the beans just before using them.
4. A burr grinder is the best for grinding beans consistently and as desired.
5. Grind the beans as recommended for the method used. For example, expresso beans should be ground very finely while pour over works best with a coarser grind.
6. For best results, weigh the beans and the water. Although this seems ritualistic to some and a lot of trouble, it leads to excellent coffee. Some enjoy the rituals associated with this approach and appreciate how it helps start their day.
7. Start with cold water, filtered, if necessary, in your location. Heat the water to the optimum temperature, generally around 195–200 degrees Fahrenheit. There are kettles available that indicate the water temperature.

8. Pay close attention to the proportions of water to coffee. Recommendations on this vary slightly, but a 1:16 ratio of coffee to water produces excellent results.

9. If brewing pour-over coffee, your decision on the method to use may involve what kind of filter you prefer. Some opt for metal filters, which work well and generate less waste than paper filters, but some dislike the slight residue that remains in the coffee with metal filters. Paper filters produce a very clean cup with no residue to affect the taste. If you use paper filters rinse the vessel out with hot water before brewing the coffee to get rid of any flavors imparted by the filter. Paper filters are not as sustainable as metal ones.

10. With pour over coffee your first pour should be about one quarter to one third of the volume and then wait 35 to 40 seconds after that to continue pouring. With freshly ground coffee the first pour, the bloom, releases carbon dioxide and enhances the flavor.

Following these suggestions will enable you to brew flavorful, pleasing coffee.

Jus Alpukat – Indonesian Coffee-Avocado Shake Two superfoods combine into one tasty shake.

1¼ cups milk (dairy or plant-based)
½ cup sweetened condensed milk (or vegan substitute*)
2 medium Hass avocados, peeled and pitted
¼ cup very strong brewed coffee (espresso is best)
Pinch of kosher salt
As needed, ice (start with about a cup and add more as needed)
As desired, chocolate syrup
Combine the milk, condensed milk, avocados, coffee, and salt in a blender. Puree well. Add the ice and blend. Adjust texture with more ice if needed.
Drizzle the interior of a tall glass with chocolate and add the avocado mixture.
*sweetened condensed coconut milk or Coco Lopez cream of coconut. You can use Vegan Coffeemate, but you will have to reduce the amount of milk in the recipe.

Coffee Images
Carroll "Coffee as Superfood"
From Wikipedia Commons: Coffee
https://upload.wikimedia.org/wikipedia/commons/b/b0/Palestinian_women_grind-ing_coffee_beans.jpg

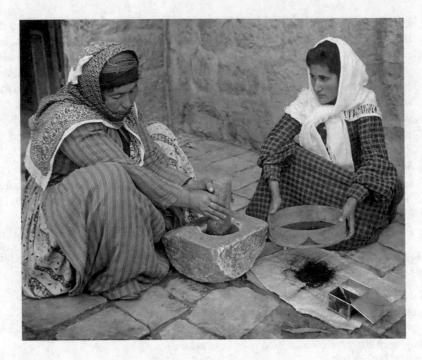

Palestinian women grinding coffee beans in 1905 (jpg)
Keystone View Company, Public domain, via Wikimedia Commons

https://upload.wikimedia.org/wikipedia/commons/f/fa/Colombian_Coffee.jpg

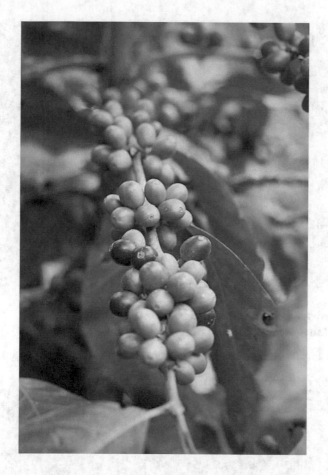

Colombian Coffee Cherries

https://upload.wikimedia.org/wikipedia/commons/4/40/Coffee_Harvesting%2C_Las_Nubes-Guatemala_MET_DP279294.jpg

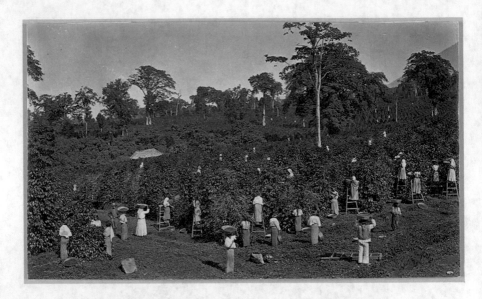

Coffee Harvesting, Las Nubes-Guatemala
Eadweard Muybridge, CC0, via Wikimedia Commons

https://upload.wikimedia.org/wikipedia/commons/f/f0/Coffee_beans_roasted.jpg

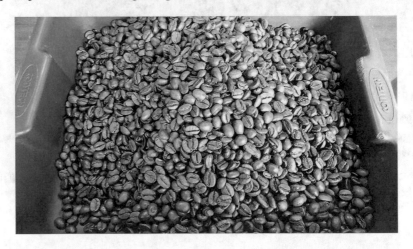

Roasted Coffee Beans
Sridhar Rao, CC BY-SA 4.0 <https://creativecommons.org/licenses/by-sa/4.0>, via
    Wikimedia Commons

https://commons.wikimedia.org/wiki/File:Coffee_Shop_Smokey.png

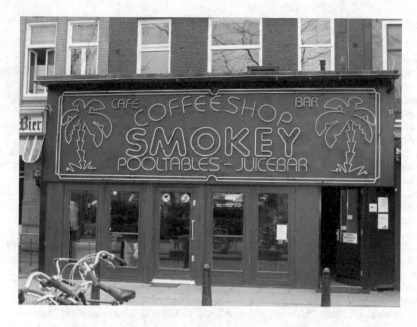

Smoky Coffee Shop in Amsterdam
Sissssou, CC BY-SA 3.0 <https://creativecommons.org/licenses/by-sa/3.0>, via
   Wikimedia Commons

https://commons.wikimedia.org/wiki/File:Royal_Armenia_Coffee.jpg

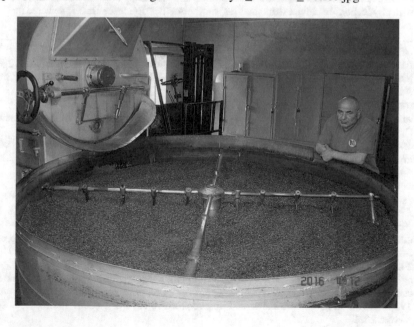

Royal Armenia Coffee
Narek75, CC BY-SA 4.0 <https://creativecommons.org/licenses/by-sa/4.0>, via
   Wikimedia Commons

References

Abe, E. L. et al. (2007). "Daily coffee consumption and prevalence of nonmelanoma skin cancer in Caucasian women." *European Journal of Cancer Prevention* 16(5):446–452. [Online]. Available at: https://doi.org/10.1097/01.cej.0000243850.59362.73. Accessed 22 May 2021

American College of Obstetricians and Gynecologists. (2020). *Moderate caffeine consumption during pregnancy*. [Online] Available at: https://www.acog.org/clinical/clinical-guidance/committee-opinion/articles/2010/08/moderate-caffeine-consumption-during-pregnancy. Accessed 21 Dec 2020.

Bamia, C., & Corenlis, M. (eds.) (2019). "The impact of caffeine and coffee on human health." Special Issue of *Nutrients*. Available at: https://www.mdpi.com/journal/nutrients/special_issues/Coffee_Caffeine_Health. Accessed 22 May 2021.

Brody, J. (2021). "Wake up to the good news about coffee." *New York Times* 14 June [online] Available at https://nytimes.com/2021/06/14/well/eat/coffee-health-benefits.html. Accessed 14 June 2021.

Cook, J. (2019). The whole-body benefits of coffee. *Consumer Reports*. November.

Dunn, R. (2017). *Never out of season: How having the food we want when we it threatens our food supply and our future*. Little, Brown.

Ellis, M. (2011). *The coffee-house: A cultural history*. Weidenfield & Nicolson.

Fridell, G. (2014). *Coffee*. Polity Press.

Grady, D. (2008). "Pregnancy problems tied to caffeine." *New York Times* 21 January [Online]. Available at: https://www.nytimes.com/2008/01/21/health/21caffeine.html. Accessed 13 Aug 2020.

Grosso, G., Godos, J., Galvano, F., & Giovannucci, E. L. (2017). Coffee, caffeine, and health outcomes: An umbrella review. *Annual Review of Nutrition, 37*, 131–156.

Harvard, T.H. Chan School of Public Health. (2021). *The Nutrition Source: Coffee*. https://www.hsph.harvard.edu/nutritionsource/food-features/coffee/. Accessed 6 May 2021.

James, J.E. (2020). "Maternal caffeine consumption and pregnancy outcomes: A narrative review with implications for advice to mothers and mothers to be." Evidence-Based Medicine (online) Available at: https://doi.org/10.1136/bmjebm-2020-111432. Accessed 11 Nov 2020.

Juma, C. (1989). *The gene hunters: Biotechnology and the scramble for seeds*. Princeton University Press.

Klatsky, P., & Tran, N. (2008). "Letter to the editor: Coffee and pregnancy" *New York Times*, 2 Feb [Online] Available at: https://www.nytimes.com/2008/02/02/opinion/lweb02pregnancy.html. Accessed 14 Jan 2021.

Morris, J. (2018). *Coffee: A global history*. Reaktion.

Pollan, M. (2019). Caffeine: How caffeine created the modern world. Audio Book. Audible Original

Saverio, et al. (2017). Coffee, tea and melanoma risk: Findings from the European prospective investigation into cancer and nutrition. *International Journal of Cancer* 140:2246–2266. (Online) Available at: https://doi.org/10.1002/ijc.30659. Accessed 15 Feb 2021.

Tucker, C. M. (2011). *Coffee culture: Local experiences, global connections*. Routledge.

Van Dam, R., Hu, F.B., & Willett, W.C. (2020 July 23). Coffee, caffeine, and health. *The New England Journal of Medicine*. 383(4):369–378. https://doi.org/10.1056/NEJMra1816604. Accessed 12 Feb 2021.

Van der Vossen, H., Bertrand, B., & Charrier, A. (2015). Next generation variety development for sustainable production of arabica coffee (Coffea arabica L.): A review. *Euphytica, 204*(2), 243–256.

Weng, X., Odouli, R., & Li, D. (2008). "Maternal caffeine consumption during pregnancy and the risk of miscarriage: a prospective cohort study." *American Journal of Obstetrics and Gynecology* 198(3):279.e1–8. [Online] Available at: https://doi.org/10.1016/j.ajog.2007.10.803. Accessed: 14 Mar 2021.

Chapter 6
Dark Leafy Greens

Marisa Bunning and Elisa Shackleton

Impressive nutritional and phytochemical profiles have helped dark leafy greens earn their super food status. Leafy vegetables improve dietary quality by providing several essential vitamins and minerals, as well as fiber, while only adding minor amounts of sodium, cholesterol, and carbohydrates. Evidence from a wide variety of research studies indicates that antioxidants found in leafy green vegetables may help protect heart health, vision, memory, and reduce the risk of cancer by protecting cells from free radical damage (AICR, 2020; Roberts & Moreau, 2016; Yan, 2016). The ability of these low-calorie standouts to bring so many benefits to our plates is proof that leafy greens are truly nutritionally-gifted vegetables.

Due to variations in pigmentation and growth stage, leafy crops range in color from light to dark green and vary in texture from delicate to quite sturdy. Several of the richly pigmented types are known as dark leafy green vegetables and will be the focus of this chapter. Five of the most popular types are collards, kale, spinach, Swiss chard, and beet greens. These greens belong to two different plant families, Brassicacae and Amaranthaceae, and their nutritional attributes are highlighted in Table 6.1.

6.1 Cultural History

The leaves of hundreds of types of herbaceous species contribute to diets around the world. Brkic et al. (2017) were able to collect 200 different types of leafy green vegetables sold in the Republic of Croatia although in some other parts of the world, only a few types are generally available. The leaves of annual plants were likely first

M. Bunning (✉) · E. Shackleton
Colorado State University, Fort Collins, CO, USA
e-mail: marisa.bunning@colostate.edu

Table 6.1 Selected nutrients per one cup of leafy greens, cooked

	Collards	Kale	Spinach	Swiss chard	Beet greens
Family	• Brassicaceae		• Amaranthaceae		
Name	*Brassica oleracea, variety acephala*	Brassica oleracea, variety acephala	*Spinacia oleracea*	*Beta vulgaris, variety cicla*	*Beta vulgaris*
Calories/100 g	32	35	41	35	39
Vit. A	100%	96%	**377%**	214%	220%
Vit. K	364%	325%	**740%**	477%	871%
Calcium	18%	**20%**	19%	8%	13%
Iron	0%	9%	**36%**	22%	15%

Bold font = highest level among these types
Cooked = boiled, drained, no salt added

discovered as native species but as their culinary value became known, seeds and plants were collected and transported to other areas. These were planted as garden herbs but over time became naturalized and eventually were grown in commercial operations. While early specimens of many vegetable crops, such as tomatoes and corn, barely resemble their relatives found in grocery stores today, the appearance of cultivated leafy vegetables has not changed noticeably compared to their wild relatives, such as dandelion greens, Lamb's Quarters, and pokeweed.

Leafy vegetables can grow well in a range of climates, at least during cooler seasons when temperatures do not exceed 85 °F (Fouladkhah et al., 2011; Westenhiser, 2020). Ease of growing and a relatively short time from planting to harvest have contributed to the cultivation of leafy green crops in almost every country in the world. Greens can be grown in a variety of settings: on farms covering hundreds of acres, in green houses, in home gardens, or in individual trays or pots. Even those of us without a 'green thumb' are able to produce a good crop of greens (Bunning et al., 2010).

Although mature stages are more familiar to us, leafy greens are now available as young baby greens and even in micro form, as microgreens. Microgreens, an emerging food crop receiving high marks for sustainability, are leafy green seedlings harvested between 10 and 14 days after germination (Michell et al., 2020). Evidence indicates these adolescent plants are higher in vitamin, mineral, and phytochemical content than their mature plant counterparts and found to be highly acceptable to consumers.

While there are similarities among leafy greens, each type has its own distinguishing characteristics.

Collards are well known for being cooked with smoked and salted pork, partly because these greens are substantial enough to hold their own with other strong flavors. Collards are associated with Southern cuisine (UIC, 2020), but they are popular across the U.S. and in many other regions of the world, including Africa, Eastern Europe, and South America. A serendipitous benefit of collards' long cooking time can be the pot likker (liquor), the nutritious liquid broth that remains after collards and other greens are cooked down (Weinzweig, 2009).

Kale has recently become a signature dish for healthy diets (Harvard, 2020; Šamec et al., 2019) and a star of the farm-to-table movement. Kale can be an acquired taste and proof of that challenge might be the popular practice of transforming kale leaves into salted, crunchy kale chips. Nutritionally, kale stands out among all types of produce for its high vitamin C content, with one serving providing more than 100% of the Daily Reference Value (DRV) based on a 2000 calorie per day diet (USDA, 2020). With variations in color, from bright green to bluish, and leaf structure that ranges from frilly to bumpy, the varietal offerings of kale are often associated with different uses. Mature kale leaves can be used in salads but often benefit from massaging or the addition of an acid, like lemon juice, to soften their somewhat tough texture (See Recipe 1, Massaged Kale). Lacinato, also called Tuscan or dinosaur kale because of its unique bumpy texture, is a traditional ingredient in minestrone. Red Russian kale and other specialty types are often sold at farmers' markets and can add color and flavor to soups and pasta dishes.

Spinach, one of the most versatile of the dark leafy greens, works equally well as a raw salad ingredient or a cooked green and is even delicate enough to be used in soufflés and dips. The association of the term 'Florentine' with dishes containing spinach reportedly dates back to the 1530s when Catherine, wife of Henry II, introduced her favorite Tuscan ingredients to France, helping to boost the popularity of this green (FLC, 2020). In the 1930s spinach gained notoriety as the source of strength of the famous cartoon character, Popeye, which led to increased consumption (Trinklein, 2020) and made it one of the first recognized super foods (Roberts & Moreau, 2016). Although exaggerated iron and Vitamin A content has reportedly been attributed to spinach because of the comic strip (Schwarcz, 2017; Sutton, 2010), cooked spinach has an impressive nutritional profile (Table 6.1). The two main types of spinach are Savoy, with crinkly leaves, and flat or smooth leaf, which is the type most often used for canning or freezing (Trinklein, 2020).

Swiss chard: the European adjective adds an air of sophistication but chard is also at home in any farmers' market or roadside stand. The word Swiss was added by producers, possibly as a tribute to a Swiss botanist, to help distinguish it from a type known as French chard (FSI 2020). Rainbow chard, with its colorful stems and earthy flavor, is especially popular. Due to its delicate texture and pleasant taste, chard is frequently used in Mediterranean cuisines for flavoring soups and pasta dishes.

Beet greens: what is not to like about a plant that gives us a richly colored edible root and tasty leaves to boot? Due to this double value and a long shelf life, beets were considered an essential winter food for the colonists and helped them to endure the 'Six Weeks of Want,' the period from end of January to mid-March, when produce was especially scarce (Smithsonian, 2020). Beet greens are often preferred by greens enthusiasts because of their sweet flavor and silky texture.

6.2 Survey of the Current State of Nutritional Research and Health Claims

Leafy greens supply many necessary nutrients including some recognized as deficient in U.S. diets. The 2015–2020 Dietary Guidelines for Americans identified calcium, iron (for certain age/gender groups), and vitamin A among the nutrients that are underconsumed in the U.S. (USDA, 2020). With their rich nutrient portfolios (Table 6.1), the 2020 Guidelines recommend consuming at least one and a half cups per week of dark green vegetables.

Evidence from a variety of research studies indicates that diets rich in fruits and vegetables are protective against common chronic diseases, such as cancer, obesity, diabetes, and cardiovascular disease (AICR, Boeing et al., 2012; Yan, 2016). Leafy green vegetables, in particular, are recognized as having substantial health-promoting activities due to the functional properties of their nutrients and protective chemical compounds (Roberts & Moreau, 2016). Their diverse nutritional composition includes vitamins, minerals, and bioactive phytochemicals that scavenge reactive oxygen species and prevent oxidative damage. This range of biological active components associated with greens contributes to their anti-cancer, anti-obesity, hypoglycemic, and hypolipidemic properties (Roberts & Moreau, 2016; Yan, 2016).

Diets rich in vegetables, as part of a western diet, have been associated with improved cognitive health (Gehlich et al., 2020). In a prospective study involving 960 older adults, approximately one serving per day of green leafy vegetables was positively and significantly associated with slower decline in brain function (Morris et al., 2018). Two bioactive compounds found in leafy greens, lutein and zeaxanthin (L + Z), function broadly in a number of brain regions, including cognition, decision-making, and visual perception (Demmig-Adams et al., 2020). Renzi-Hammond et al. (2017) also reported supplementation with L + Z improved spatial memory, reasoning ability, and complex attention in young, healthy adults. These two carotenoids are also known to filter harmful blue wavelengths of light which helps protect and maintain healthy cells in the eyes (AOA, 2020). Of the hundreds of carotenoids found in nature, only L + Z are uniquely concentrated in the retina and lens, indicating that both perform vital functions in these ocular tissues (Mares, 2016). Research supports the view that these phytochemicals have a potential role in the prevention and treatment of certain eye diseases, such as age-related macular degeneration, cataracts, and retinitis pigmentos (AOA, 2020). The American Optometric Association (2020) reports that the level of L + Z associated with health benefit is 6 mg per day (Table 6.2).

Gluocosinolates are sulfur-containing compounds that are broken down into iso-thiocyanates and indole-3-carbinol during cooking and digestion. Laboratory

Table 6.2 Lutein + Zeaxanthin per one cup of leafy greens, cooked

	Collards	Kale	Spinach	Swiss chard	Beet greens
Lutein + Zeaxanthin	4.323 mg	6.261 mg	20.354 mg	19.276 mg	2.619 mg

research has shown these compounds protect healthy cells and observational studies have suggested a protective effect on cardiovascular health and certain types of cancer but more work is needed to understand the role of various bioactive molecules (Harvard, 2020).

6.2.1 Greens and Anti-nutrients

Despite the many associated health benefits, leafy greens also produce certain compounds that have been associated with potentially negative health impacts. The organic acid, oxalate, is naturally synthesized by humans but also produced by plants, including leafy vegetables. Beet greens, spinach (raw and cooked), and collard greens tend to be high in oxalates while kale has a relatively low level (Univ. Chicago, 2020). The consumption of additional oxalate has been linked to the formation of kidney stones and other health issues because oxalate binds with calcium and other minerals (Noonan & Savage, 1999). Dietary nitrates, which are present in leafy greens, have been associated with increased incidence of cancer (Lidder & Webb, 2013) however, several studies have reported positive health impacts of habitual dietary nitrate intake. An Australian study (n = 3759) comparing intake of nitrate-containing foods and muscle function provided evidence of long-term benefits of nitrate intake obtained primarily from vegetables (Sim et al., 2021). A separate Australian study demonstrated an inverse relationship between vegetable nitrate intake and cardiovascular disease among an older population of men and women (Liu et al., 2018). Bondonno et al. (2021) reported that moderate to high nitrate intakes from vegetables were associated with lower risk of ischemic heart disease, peripheral artery disease, ischemic stroke, and heart failure among 53,150 participants of the Danish Diet, Cancer, and Health Study.

> Another concern is related to the goitrogen content in Kale and other greens. These substances can block iodine from Dark leafy greens and anti-nutrients reaching the thyroid gland and may increase the risk of goiter (Harvard, 2020).

6.3 Survey of the Botany, Biology, and Chemistry of Leafy Greens

6.3.1 The Complex Life of Leaves

Leafy greens are composed of tissues that are fundamentally different from the harvested portion of other fruit and vegetable crops (Evert & Eichhorn, 2013). Botanically speaking, fruits are seed-containing tissues of plants, which are designed to protect and provide nourishment for the germinated seeds. Vegetables, however, are derived from other parts of plants, such as tap roots (carrots), fleshy stalks (celery), and tubers (potatoes), with their primary function being storage of carbohydrates, nutrients, and water. In contrast to fruits and other types of vegetables, the primary job of leaves is photosynthesis and that function is closely associated with their morphology. Leaves are generally flat, thin, and densely packed with chloroplasts to maximize surface area and increase their potential to intercept light. Leafy vegetables tend to be formed into dense rosettes around a central axis which magnifies their ability to photosynthesize, in other words, to convert light and carbon dioxide into glucose and oxygen.

6.3.2   The Need to Be Green

Pigments in leaves are synthesized in response to light and provide an effective protective screen because they absorb light from 280 to 340 nm in wavelength but do not diminish the amount of photosynthetically active radiation, which ranges from 400 to 700 nm (ALL, 2020). The pigments which give leafy crops their characteristic color are classified as porphyrins (chlorophylls), carotenoids (carotenes, xanthophylls), flavonoids (anthocyanins, flavonols, flavones) or phenolics (tannins, lignin) (Evert & Eichhorn, 2013).

6.3.3   Induced Defense Weapons

In addition to being the site of light-catching infrastructure, leaves are accumulation areas for various phytochemicals with antioxidant, light-filtering, antimicrobial, antiherbivorial, and other defensive properties (Tarwadi & Agte, 2003). Unlike members of the animal kingdom, plants rely on a 'chemical defense system' to compensate for their inability to evade threats, such as insects, plant pathogens, and intense radiation. Consequently, leafy vegetables are particularly good sources of bioactive compounds. By necessity, leaves are complex systems with enzymatic, physiochemical, microbiological, and defense mechanisms occurring simultaneously (Evert & Eichhorn, 2013). Within plant leaves, oxygen molecules act as electron acceptors for photosynthesis and as substrates in photorespiration. These processes produce a number of reactive oxygen species, including hydrogen peroxide and hydroxyl radicals. As a result, plant cells have embraced the potential for using oxygen for metabolism while limiting the deleterious effects of oxygen interactions by producing a variety of antioxidants (Evert & Eichhorn, 2013; Lobo et al., 2010). The biochemical production necessary for photosynthesis and plant defense accounts for their distinctive tastes compared to other produce. Greens are low in sweetness, often even bitter, but very enjoyable – and healthy choices for us!

6.4 Sustainability, Environmental Health Concerns, Agricultural Issues, Fair Trade and Marketing Issues of Greens

In terms of nutrition and dietary benefits, leafy greens are standout vegetables but there are several challenges associated with their production, pre-harvest and post-harvest. Even though they are low on the scale of water required for production of food crops (Mekonnen & Hoekstra, 2010), leafy greens are shallow-rooted crops that need frequent irrigation throughout the growing season. This makes them particularly sensitive to drought stress and inconsistent watering can result in undesirable texture and appearance (CAFE, 2020). Their vulnerability to temperatures in the 90s is another climatic factor that is challenging for producers.

The post-harvest period can be problematic with vegetables because after harvest plants cells continue to respire, that is utilize stored reserves and release carbon dioxide. Leaves tend to exhibit a rapid rate of respiration, making leafy vegetables a highly perishable food item. Even with refrigeration and careful handling, the shelf life of all leafy greens is fairly short and environmental conditions, such as temperature and humidity, have large impacts on storage time and quality.

In spite of these challenges, leafy green vegetables also have several important production advantages. While many types of produce with reputations as super foods require tropical climatic conditions for optimum growth, leafy greens can be quite easy to grow so they are cultivated around the globe. And unlike most fruits and vegetables, such as peaches or tomatoes, the flavor of greens is not dependent on maturity or ripeness. In fact, young leaves are often preferred for their taste and texture. For this reason, growing periods can be as short as three weeks for the immature leaves known as 'baby greens.' Leafy vegetable crops are planted annually and classified as cool season crops but they are capable of growing under many different environmental conditions. Leafy crops undergo dramatic changes when temperatures rise above the mid-eighties, changing from rosette leaf formations to tall plants with elongated internodes and terminal flowers, a process referred to as bolting. As plants shift their resources to support seed production, sugar content of leaves decreases, resulting in amplified bitterness (Evert & Eichhorn, 2013). Bolting can greatly reduce the quality and value of a leafy crop.

6.4.1 Unintentional Vehicles for Pathogens

Ironically, in spite of their numerous health benefits, leafy greens can inadvertently be carriers of harmful microorganisms. Their high surface area and proximity to soil make leafy greens vulnerable to bacterial contamination and unfortunately, they have been the source of many foodborne illness outbreaks (Appold, 2019). Contamination can occur at any step in the supply chain and is difficult, if not impossible, to remove (FDA, 2020). This complex and recurring problem for leafy greens is primarily linked with those that are consumed raw, such as lettuce. Dark leafy greens are often cooked which reduces the risk of illness although some types, including spinach and kale, are frequently consumed without cooking. Following safe handling practices is critical from farm to table to reduce this risk (Bunning & Kendall, 2012).

6.5   Culinary Uses

It should be noted that consuming leafy greens can become habit forming. Although their flavor is often referred to as bitter, this can be a positive attribute and may be one of the reasons behind collards' and kale's enthusiastic following. They can become one of those foods you start to crave – you may recall that Rapunzel's woes started with her mother's insatiable craving for the fresh green that grew only in the witch's garden (Ashliman, 2013). Greens also seem to have a strong connection to memory – they may remind you of your grandmother's kitchen (Harris, 1998) or trips to New Orleans, Savannah, or Italy. Although more commonly seen as a side dish than an entree, dark leafy greens add supportive complexity to main dishes – for example spinach to quiche, kale to bean soup, chard to lasagna, and arugula to pizza.

Preparation Tips   The texture of stems or midribs of leafy greens can be much tougher than the thinner blade sections making it necessary to 'destem' before cooking. This can be done by folding the leaf in half and cutting next to the stem or pulling the leaf through a specially designed destemming tool.

- The stalks can be eaten but should be cooked separately from leaves since they may take longer to cook.
- Be warned, what starts out looking like a large mess of greens can end up being a piddling amount. Since water is a major component in leaves, the cooking process releases that water from cells, greatly changing the texture and cooking volume.

6.6   Give the Green Light to These Recipes

Massaged Kale Salad with Lemon and Garlic   This salad calls for a unique physical approach, which not only improves the texture but also helps to reduce bitterness.

Serves: 4
Ingredients:

- 2–3 tablespoons lemon juice
- 1–2 cloves garlic, crushed or finely minced

- 1 bunch of green curly or lacinato kale, washed, stemmed, and cut into thin strips
- 3 tablespoons olive oil
- 1/4 cup parmesan cheese, finely shredded (optional)
- 1/4 cup roasted nuts of choice, chopped (optional)
- Salt and pepper, to taste

Directions:

1. In a small bowl, combine crushed/minced garlic and lemon juice. Set aside.
2. In a large bowl, add kale, and cover with olive oil. Using your clean hands, massage the oil into the kale until the leaves soften and turn a darker green, about 1–2 minutes.
3. Pour lemon and garlic mixture over kale, toss to coat.
4. Add salt and pepper to taste.
5. Top salad with parmesan cheese and roasted nuts, if desired.

Spanish Greens

2 Tablespoons olive oil
3 cloves garlic, flattened or smashed with the flat of a knife
1 pound spinach, chard, collards or other greens, stemmed and well washed
Salt and pepper to taste
¼ cup golden raisins
3 Tablespoons toasted pine nuts

Heat oil over high heat in a very large skillet. Add garlic cloves and stir-fry until golden, about 30 seconds Discard garlic. Toss in greens. Season with salt and pepper. Cover; wilt greens 2–3 minutes. Add raisins and pine nuts. Check for seasoning and serve. Makes 2–4 servings.

From Asparagus to Zucchini: A Guide to Cooking Farm-Fresh Seasonal Produce, 3rd Edition: FairShare CSA Coalition, Wubben, Doug: 9780615230139.

http://foodsmartcolorado.colostate.edu/2020/04/14/massaged-kale-with-garlic-and-lemon/

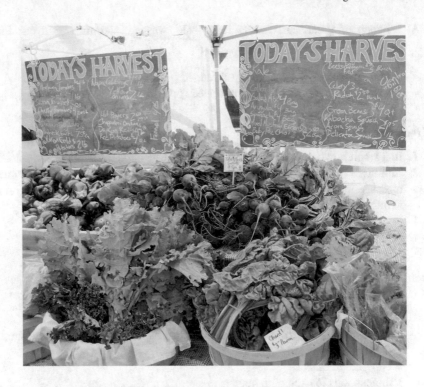

Photo by Colorado State University Extension Service. Used by permission.

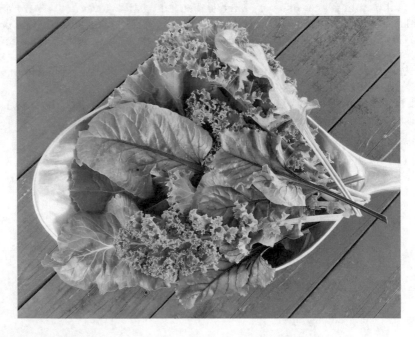

Photo by Colorado State University Extension Service. Used by permission.

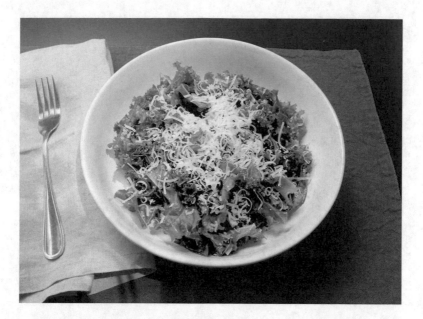

Photo by Colorado State University Extension Service. Used by permission.

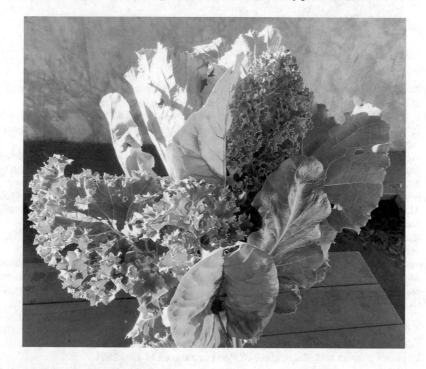

Photo by Colorado State University Extension Service. Used by permission.

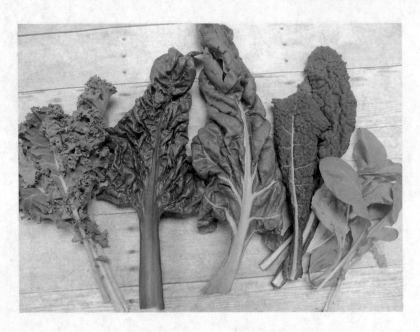

Photo by Colorado State University Extension Service. Used by permission.

References

AICR. (2020). *Foods that fight cancer, American Institute for Cancer Research* [Online]. Available at: https://www.aicr.org/cancer-prevention/food-facts/. Accessed 10 Dec 2020.

ALL. (2020). *The light-dependent reactions of photosynthesis, affordable learning louis biology 2e* [Online]. Available at: https://louis.oercommons.org/courseware/module/638/student/?task=3. Accessed 12 Dec 2020.

AOA. (2020). *Diet and nutrition: Adding powerful antioxidants to your diet can improve your eye health/American Optometric Association* [Online]. Available at: https://www.aoa.org/healthy-eyes/caring-for-your-eyes/diet-and-nutrition?sso=y. Accessed 6 Dec 2020.

Appold, K. (2019). Challenges of preventing leafy green outbreaks, *Food Quality and Safety* (June 11, 2019) [Online]. Available at: https://www.foodqualityandsafety.com/article/fresh-produce-outbreaks-challenges-prevention/. Accessed 6 Dec 2020.

Ashliman, D.L. (2013). *Grimm Brothers' Home Page, University of Pittsburgh* [Online]. Available at: https://www.pitt.edu/~dash/grimm.html. Accessed 20 Dec 2020.

Boeing, H., Bechthold, A., Bub, A., Ellinger, S., Haller, D., Kroke, A., Leschik-Bonnet, E., Muller, M., Oberritter, H., Schulze, M., Stehle, P., & Watzl, B. (2012). Critical review: vegetables and fruit in the prevention of chronic diseases. *European Journal of Nutrition, 51*(6), 637–663.

Bondonno, C.P., Dalgaard, F., Blekkenhorst, L.C., Murray, K., Lewis, J.R., Croft, K.D., Kyro, C., Torp-Pedersen, C., Gislason, G., Tjonneland, A., Overvad, K., Bondonno, N., & Hodgson, J.M. (2021). Vegetable nitrate intake, blood pressure and incident cardiovascular disease: Danish diet, cancer, and health study, *European Journal of Epidemiology*. [Online] Available at: https://pubmed.ncbi.nlm.nih.gov/33884541/. Accessed 14 June 2021.

Brkić, D., Bošnir, J., Bevardi, M., Bošković, A. G., Miloš, S., Lasić, D., Krivohlavek, A., Racz, A., Ćuić, A. M., & Trstenjak, N. U. (2017). Nitrate in leafy green vegetables and estimated intake. *African Journal of Traditional, Complementary, and Alternative Medicines, 14*(3), 31–41.

Bunning, M., & Kendall, P. (2012). *Health benefits and safe handling of salad greens, Colorado State University Extension* [Online]. Available at: https://extension.colostate.edu/topic-areas/ nutrition-food-safety-health/health-benefits-and-safe-handling-of-salad-greens-9-373/. Accessed 13 Dec 2020.

Bunning, M., Stonaker, F., & Card, A. (2010) *Growing container salad greens, Colorado State University Extension* [Online]. Available at: https://extension.colostate.edu/topic-areas/ nutrition-food-safety-health/growing-container-salad-greens-9-378/. Accessed 16 Nov 2020.

CAFE. (2020). *Irrigating vegetable crops, The Center for Agriculture, Food, and the Environment, University of Massachusetts Amherst Extension Vegetable Program* [Online]. Available at: https://ag.umass.edu/vegetable/fact-sheets/irrigating-vegetable-crops. Accessed 15 Dec 2020.

Demmig-Adams, B., López-Pozo, M., Stewart, J. J., & Adams, W. W. (2020). Zeaxanthin and lutein: Photoprotectors, anti-inflammatories, and brain food. *Molecules, 25*(16) [Online] Available at: https://pubmed.ncbi.nlm.nih.gov/32784397/. Accessed 12 Dec 2020.

Evert, R., & Eichhorn, S. (2013). *Raven biology of plants* (8th ed.). W.H. Freeman and Company.

FDA. (2020). *Foodborne pathogens, U. S. Food and Drug Administration* [Online]. Available at: https://www.fda.gov/food/outbreaks-foodborne-illness/foodborne-pathogens. Accessed 14 Dec 2020

FLC. (2020). *Spinach – The Green Wonder, Food Literacy Center* [Online] Available at: https:// www.foodliteracycenter.org/. Accessed 12 Dec 2020.

Fouladkhah, A., Bunning, M., Stone, M., Stushnoff, C., Stonaker, F., & Kendall, P. (2011). Consumer hedonic evaluation of eight fresh specialty leafy greens and their relationship to instrumental quality attributes and indicators of secondary metabolites. *Journal of Sensory Science, 26*(3), 175–183.

Gehlich, K. H., Beller, J., Lange-Asschenfeldt, B., Köcher, W., Meinke, M. C., & Lademann, J. (2020). Consumption of fruits and vegetables: improved physical health, mental health, physical functioning and cognitive health in older adults from 11 European countries. *Aging & Mental Health, 24*(4), 634–641.

Harris, J. (1998). In a leaf of collard, green. In M. Winegardner (Ed.), *We are what we ate* (1st ed.). Harcourt, Brace, and Company.

Harvard University. (2020). *The nutrition source: Kale, T.H. Chan School of Public Health* [Online]. Available at: https://www.hsph.harvard.edu/nutritionsource/food-features/kale/. Accessed 15 Nov 2020.

Lidder, S., & Webb, A. J. (2013). Vascular effects of dietary nitrate (as found in green leafy vegetables and beetroot) via the nitrate-nitrite-nitric oxide pathway. *British Journal of Clinical Pharmacology, 75*(3), 677–696.

Liu, A. H., Bondonno, C. P., Russell, J., Flood, V. M., Lewis, J. R., Croft, K. D., Woodman, R. J., Lim, W. H., Kifley, A., Wong, G., Mitchell, P., Hodgson, J. M., & Blekkenhorst, L. C. (2018). Relationship of dietary nitrate intake from vegetables with cardiovascular disease mortality: A prospective study in a cohort of older Australians. *European Journal of Nutrition, 58*, 2741–2753.

Lobo, V., Patil, A., Phatak, A., & Chandra, N. (2010). 'Free radicals, antioxidants and functional foods: Impact on human health', Pharmacognosy Reviews, 4(8). [Online] Available at: https:// doi.org/10.4103/0973-7847.70902. Accessed 10 Nov 2020.

Mares, J. (2016). Lutein and zeaxanthin isomers in eye health and disease. *Annual Review of Nutrition, 36*, 571–602.

Mekonnen, M.M., & Hoekstra, A.Y. (2010). *The Green, Blue and Grey Water Footprint of Crops and Derived Crop Products, Main Report, Institute for Water Education* [Online]. Available at: https://www.waterfootprint.org/media/downloads/Report47-WaterFootprintCrops-Vol1.pdf. Accessed 30 Nov 2020.

Michell, K. A., Isweiri, H., Newman, S. E., Bunning, M., Bellows, L. L., Dinges, M. M., Grabos, L. E., Rao, S., Foster, M. T., Heuberger, A. L., Prenni, J. E., Thompson, H. J., Uchanski, M. E., Weir, T. L., & Johnson, S. A. (2020). Microgreens: consumer sensory perception and acceptance of an emerging functional food crop. *Journal of Food Science, 85*(4), 926–935.

Morris M.C., Wang Y., Barnes L.L., Bennett D.A., Dawson-Hughes B., & Booth S.L. (2018). 'Nutrients and bioactives in green leafy vegetables and cognitive decline: Prospective study', *Neurology, 90*(3) [online] Available at https://doi.org/10.1212/WNL.0000000000004815. Accessed 15 Nov 2020.

Noonan, S. C., & Savage, G. P. (1999). Oxalate content of foods and its effect on humans. *Asia Pacific Journal of Clinical Nutrition, 8*(1), 64–74.

Renzi-Hammond, L. M., Bovier, E. R., Fletcher, L. M., Miller, L. S., Mewborn, C. M., Lindbergh, C. A., Baxter, J. H., & Hammond, B. R. (2017). Effects of a lutein and zeaxanthin intervention on cognitive function: a randomized, double-masked, placebo-controlled trial of younger healthy adults [Online]. *Nutrients, 9*(11). https://doi.org/10.3390/nu9111246. Accessed 20 Nov 2020.

Roberts, J.L., & Moreau R. (2016) 'Functional properties of spinach (Spinacia oleracea L.) phytochemicals and bioactives'. Food & Function 7(8) [online]. Available at: https://doi.org/10.1039/c6fo00051g. Accessed 15 Nov 2020.

Šamec, D., Urlić, B., & Salopek-Sondi, B. (2019). Kale (*Brassica oleracea* var. *acephala*) as a superfood: review of the scientific evidence behind the statement. *Critical Reviews in Food Science and Nutrition, 59*(15) [Online]. Available at: https://pubmed.ncbi.nlm.nih.gov/29557674/. Accessed 12 Dec 2020.

Schwarcz, J. (2017). Iron in Spinach. Office for Science and Society, McGill University, https://www.mcgill.ca/oss/article/food-health-news-quirky-science/setting-facts-straight-about-iron-spinach#:~:text=Hamblin's%20theme%20was%20how%20%E2%80%9Cfrauds,handedly%20raised%20the%20consumption%20of. Accessed 12 Dec 2020.

Sim, M., Blekkenhorst, L.C., Bondonno, N.P., Radavelli-Bagatini, S., Peeling, P., Bondonno, C.P., Magliano, D.J., Shaw, J., Woodman, R., Murray, K., Lewis, J.R., Daly, R., & Hodgson, J.M. (2021). Dietary nitrate intake is positively associated with muscle function in men and women independent of physical activity levels. *The Journal of Nutrition* 151(5) [Online]. Available at: https://europepmc.org/article/med/33760920. Accessed 14 June 2021.

Smithsonian National Museum of American History. (2020). Beauty and the beets. https://americanhistory.si.edu/ja/blog/2012/06/beauty-and-the-beets.html. Accessed 28 Oct 2020.

Sutton, M. (2010). Spinach, iron and Popeye: ironic lessons from biochemistry and history on the importance of healthy eating, healthy skepticism and adequate citation. *Internet Journal of Criminology*. Available at: https://www5.in.tum.de/persons/huckle/Sutton_Spinach_Iron_and_Popeye_March_2010.pdf. Accessed 12 Dec 2020.

Tarwadi, K., & Agte, V. (2003). Potential of commonly consumed green leafy vegetables for their antioxidant capacity and its linkage with the micronutrient profile. *International Journal of Food Sciences and Nutrition, 54*, 417–425.

Trinklein, D. (2020). Spinach: Vegetable made famous by Popeye. University of Missouri Integrated Pest Management, https://ipm.missouri.edu/. Accessed 7 Dec 2020.

UIC. (2020). University of Illinois Chicago Heritage Garden: Collard Greens. Available at: http://heritagegarden.uic.edu/collard-greens-brassica-oleracea. Accessed 15 Dec 2020.

University of Chicago. (2020). How to Eat a Low Oxalate Diet. https://kidneystones.uchicago.edu/how-to-eat-a-low-oxalate-diet/. Accessed 16 Dec 2020.

USDA. (2020). U.S. Department of Agriculture, Agricultural Research Service. Food Data Central, 2020. Available at: fdc.nal.usda.gov. Accessed 12 Nov 2020.

Weinzweig, A. (2009). Potlikker: From slave plantations to today. *The Atlantic*. Available at: https://www.theatlantic.com/health/archive/2009/04/potlikker-from-slave-plantations-to-today/7129/. Accessed 22 Mar 2021.

Westenhiser, T. (2020). Swiss Chard, Food Source Information, Colorado State University [Online]. Available at: https://fsi.colostate.edu/swiss-chard/. Accessed 20 Dec 2020.

Yan, L. (2016). *Dark green leafy vegetables*. Grand Forks Human Nutrition Research Center, United States Department of Agriculture Research Service [online]. Available at: https://www.ars.usda.gov/research/publications/publications-at-this-location/?modeCode=30-62-05-00. Accessed 11 Dec 2020.

Chapter 7
Cultured Milk

Dawnie Andrak, Danielle Jacques, and Annika Weber

The universal desirability of milk is seen in ancient religions and through folklore and myth. In Greco-Roman mythology, for example, milk was the elixir of immortality. Jacopo Tintoretto's 1575 painting *The Origin of the Milky Way* depicts the moment at which Juno awakens to Hercules, her illegitimate infant son, suckling at her breast in order to obtain the gift of immortality from her milk. While Jupiter holds the baby, the tiny droplets of milk spray heavenward creating the ethereal Milky Way (Valenze, 2011) (Fig. 7.1).

Humans began fermenting milk shortly after the advent of animal domestication, beginning with goats and sheep around 8500 BCE followed by larger ruminants like cattle (7000–6000 BCE) (Chen et al., 2010, 5) and water buffalos (5000–4000 BCE) (Barker, 2014, 7696). The subtropical climate of Persia and Anatolia, with consistent temperatures of about 40°C (optimal for bacterial culture growth), likely resulted in wild, uncontrolled fermentation of stored milk and the proliferation of thickened, sour milk foodstuffs similar to yogurt (Fisberg & Machado, 2015, 5). Lactic acid fermentation extended the viability of this valuable nutrient while decreasing toxicity and increasing digestibility of the milk through the conversion of lactose into lactic acid (Laudan, 2015, 28). Given that the gene mutation for lactase persistence did not occur until roughly 5500 BCE among dairy farmers in central Europe (Itan et al., 2009, 8), some believe that dairying practices developed to meet demand for fermented rather than fresh milk (Kindstedt, 2012, 10).

D. Andrak
California State University, Sacramento, CA, USA

D. Jacques (✉)
Boston University, Boston, MA, USA
e-mail: djacques@bu.edu

A. Weber
Colorado State University, Fort Collins, CO, USA

© The Author(s), under exclusive license to Springer Nature Switzerland AG 2022
J. P. Miller, C. Van Buiten (eds.), *Superfoods*, Food and Health,
https://doi.org/10.1007/978-3-030-93240-4_7

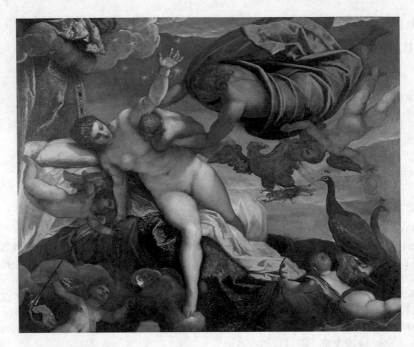

Fig. 7.1 Jacopo Tintoretto's The Origin of the Milky Way. (Photo copyright, National Gallery, London/Art Resource, New York)

Over several millennia, as dairy pastoralists migrated from the Fertile Crescent, milk consumption spread throughout the Middle East and into Central and South Asia, Southeastern Europe, Africa, Scandinavia, and the British Isles (Mlekuž, 2015, 42). Dairy fermentation techniques and traditions followed, resulting in a vast array of milk products varying in taste, texture, type of milk, microbial culture, age, acidity, and more. In the Middle East and along the eastern Mediterranean, yogurt and fresh, briny cheeses like Feta became and remain widespread. In temperate regions of Europe, cooler climates allowed dairy farmers to develop aging techniques that resulted in cheeses of all sizes, from Chabichou in France to Gruyère in Switzerland. European colonial expansion brought cheese making to the Americas, Australia, and India (Sen, 2015, 211).

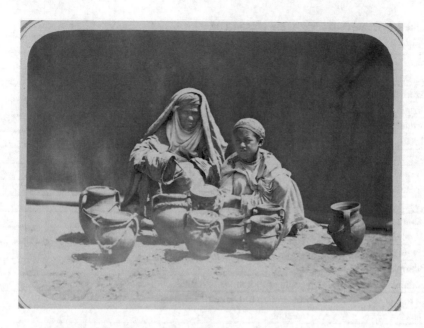

Yogurt vendors in Russian Turkestan, 1865–1872. (Illustration in Turkestan Album, Ethnographic Part, 1872, part 2, volume 2, plate 141, no. 438)

Today, fermented milk products can be found around the globe (Table 7.1). In Mongolia, pastoralists ferment mare's milk to make *airag* and *arkhi*, a milk brandy with an alcohol content as high as 18% (Turnbull, 2012, 128). During Ramadan in countries like Algeria and Iraq, Muslims break their fast in the evening with a date and a glass of *lben*, a diluted yogurt drink (Ji-Young Park, 2011, 22). *Jocoque*, derived from the Nahuatl word for "sour" (xoco), is a thickened milk seasoned with herbs and vegetables; its origins likely lie with the Arab Moors, whose culinary traditions reached Mexico by way of Spain (Abarca, 2013, 253).

7.1   The Elixir of Life Meets the Apostle of Longevity

For nearly as long as humans have consumed fermented milk, we have believed in its health benefits. Vedic texts mention a number of health benefits associated with *dadhi* (*dahi* in Hindu), a fermented milk product similar to yogurt, as early as 5000 BC (Mudgal, 2017, 353). These texts, which formed the foundation of Hinduism, considered milk and curds "immortal nectar" as they were derived from the sacred cow (Wiley, 2014, 58). Genghis Khan is reputed to have fed the Mongol army yogurt based on the belief that it would instill bravery in his soldiers (Fisberg & Machado, 2015, 5). In the eleventh century, nomadic Turks used yogurt to treat a variety of ailments like stomach cramps and sunburn, and believed in yogurt consumption's ability to prolong life (Ozen & Dinleyici, 2015, 162). By some accounts,

Table 7.1 Fermented milk products of the world

Country	Product
Armenia	matzoon, katyk, tan
Central Asia	chal, shubat, chalap, kumis, qatyq, qurt, suzma, ayran, kaymak
Azerbaijan	dovga, ayran
Bosnia and Herzegovina	kiselo mlijeko and kefir
Brittany	laezh-ribod or lait ribot
Brazil	iogurte, coalhada
Bulgaria	kiselo mlyako
Burundi	urubu
Croatia	mileram/kiselo vrhnje
Czech Republic	kefír or acidofilní mléko
Denmark	kærnemælk, tykmælk, and ymer
Dominican Republic	boruga
Estonia	soured milk and kefir
Ethiopia	ergo
Finland	piimä, viili, kotijuusto, rahka
Germany	Sauermilch or Dickmilch, Quark
Georgia	matsoni
Greece	xinogalo or xinogala (ξινόγαλα), ariani (αριάνι), kefiri (κεφίρι)
Hungary	aludttej, joghurt, kefir, tejföl
Iceland	skyr, súrmjólk, sýrður rjómi
India	dahi, lassi, chaas or Moru, mattha, mishti doi and shrikhand
Indonesia	dadiah
Iran	doogh, kashk, ghara
Kurdistan Region	mastaw
Latvia	skābais krējums
Japan	calpis, Yakult
Kenya	Kule Naoto, Maziwa Lala, Mursik, Amabere amaruranu
Latvia	rūgušpiens, kefīrs, paniņas, lakto
Lebanon	labneh, zabedi
Lithuania	rūgpienis, kefyras, grietinė
Macedonia	kiselo mleko
Mexico	jocoque, crema espesa
Mongolia	airag, arkhi byaslag, tarag, khuruud
Netherlands	karnemelk (buttermilk), drinkyoghurt
Nicaragua	leche agria
Norway	surmelk or kulturmelk, kefir, and tjukkmjølk, rømme
Pakistan	dahi and lassi
Poland	twaróg, kwaśna śmietana
Portugal	coalhada
Romania	lapte bătut, lapte acru, kefir, sana, smântână

(continued)

Table 7.1 (continued)

Country	Product
Russia, Ukraine, Belarus	kefir, prostokvasha, ryazhenka, varenets, tvorog, acidophiline, smetana
Rwanda	kivuguto
Saudi Arabia	leben, raib
Scotland	blaand
Serbia	kiselo mleko, kisela pavlaka
Slovakia	kefír, acidofilné mlieko, smotana
Slovenia	kislo mleko
South Africa	amasi (maas in Afrikaans)
Sudan	rob
Sweden	filmjölk, långfil and A-fil, grädddfil
Syria	Doogh, kashk
Tanzania	Maziwa Mgando, Maziwa Mtindi, Samli
Turkic countries	ayran, qatiq, kefir, yogurt, kımız
United States	clabber, sour cream
Zambia	mabisi
Zimbabwe	lacto

Adapted from Wikipedia
En.wikipedia.org. (n.d.) *Fermented milk products – Wikipedia*. [Online] Available at: https://en.wikipedia.org/wiki/Fermented_milk_products. Accessed 24 Oct 2020

it was considered by medieval Turks to be the elixir of life (Gasbarrini et al., 2016, 117).

European scientists began "rationalizing" these health claims in the mid nineteenth century, with Louis Pasteur's identification of microorganisms in the process of fermentation in 1857 and Joseph Lister's discovery of lactic acid fermentation in 1873 (Aryana & Olson, 2017, 9987). In 1905, a Bulgarian graduate student named Stamen Grigoroff discovered the microbe responsible for curdling milk (later naming it *Lactobacillus bulgaricus* in honor of his home country) while analyzing a yogurt sample from his hometown. Grigoroff was invited to present his findings at the Pasteur Institute, where Nobel laureate and "apostle of longevity" Ilya Mechnikov was studying the relationship between gut bacteria and aging. Mechnikov believed toxic microorganisms in the colon caused aging and deterioration of the body through "autointoxication," a theory that developed in tandem with widespread intestinal problems in over-crowded European cities (Stoilova, 2015, 19). Building on Grigoroff's discovery, Mechnikov anecdotally connected yogurt to the longevity of Bulgarian peasants who consumed it daily. He published his theory of yogurt's anti-aging capabilities in *The Prolongation of Life* (1908), "proving" yogurt's mystical health properties.

Mechnikov's acclaim helped bring this previously obscure foodstuff from the fringes of Europe to health-conscious consumers of Western Europe and beyond. In 1919, a Sephardic immigrant named Isaac Carasso founded Danone yogurt brand in Barcelona, according to the company website, after observing Spanish children suffering from intestinal infections (Danone, 2021). Later, his son moved operations to Paris and began selling ceramic yogurt containers in French pharmacies. Inspired by Mechnikov, microbiologist Minoru Shirota isolated *Lactobacillus casei* in 1930 and introduced a fermented milk beverage, Yakult, to Japan in 1935 (Yotova, 2018, 51). The history of Mechnikov's research tying Bulgarian longevity to yogurt consumption still remains an important selling point for Meiji Bulgaria Yogurt, Japan's largest yogurt producer (Meiji Co Ltd., 2020). Similarly, Indonesia-based KIN Yogurt describes yogurt as a "miracle food" and claims that "Bulgaria undoubtedly has the most beautiful people in the world" due to the youth-sustaining properties of yogurt (KIN Yogurt, 2021).

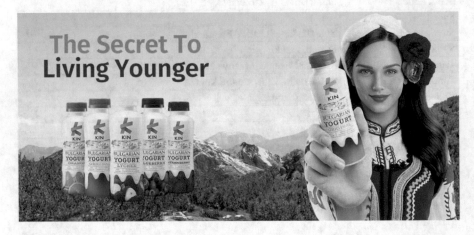

KIN Yogurt advertisement ties traditional Bulgarian yogurt to longevity. (**https://www.kindairy. com/en/kin-yogurt**)

7.2   Health Benefits of Fermented Milk

Milk is a first life-sustaining food. By definition, milk is a bodily secretion of female mammals. Mammalian milk is often referred to as "True Milk."[1] It is passed from mother to young and supplies nutrition and immunological protection. It performs

---

[1] There are a few animals that produce what is sometimes referred to as "false milk." Among them are pigeons, flamingos, and emperor penguins that produce a milky coop called "crop milk" (named so because it is produced in the bird's crop). Additionally, there is a long-standing legal debate over the definition of "milk," particularly in the United States. According to the United States Federal Drug Administration, "*Milk* means the lacteal secretion, practically free from colostrum, obtained by the complete milking of one or more healthy cows, which may be clarified and may be adjusted by separating part of the fat there from; concentrated milk, reconstituted milk, and dry whole milk. Water, in a sufficient quantity to reconstitute concentrated and dry forms, may be added." This definition and, specifically its lack of enforcement as it relates to items such as Rice Milk, Almond Milk, Oat Milk, etc., has been legally visited and revisited a number of times in recent years alone much to the chagrin of dairy farmers who would like to hold the title "milk" strictly for their product. A discussion for another paper.

these functions with a large array of distinctive compounds. While there is some variation across species, mammalian milk is a resource for lipids, proteins, amino acids, vitamins and minerals. It contains immunoglobulins, hormones, growth factors, cytokines, nucleotides, peptides, polyamines, enzymes and other bioactive peptides. All of this makes milk a nutrient-rich food that may promote positive health effects (Haug et al., 2007).

Fermentation, by definition, is the process by which microorganisms or enzymes act on food raw materials and in turn create biochemical changes (Geissler and Powers 2011, 34). Milk fermentation primarily utilizes lactic acid fermentation via lactic acid bacteria (LAB). Yeasts and molds may also be used along with LAB depending on the fermented milk product as they provide additional flavors and textures. LAB used in milk fermentation can be roughly categorized into two groups depending on their optimum growth temperature: thermophilic (30°C to 45°C) and mesophilic (20°C to 30°C). Traditionally, owing to these optimum growth temperatures, warmer regions such as the Middle East and Greece fermented their milk products with thermophilic LAB, while cooler regions such as Northern Europe depended on mesophilic LAB (Wouters et al., 2002, 92). Most industries now inoculate milk with an assortment of starter cultures rather than using traditional methods of spontaneous fermentation, which is slower and less uniform (Leroy & De Vuyst, 2004, 69).

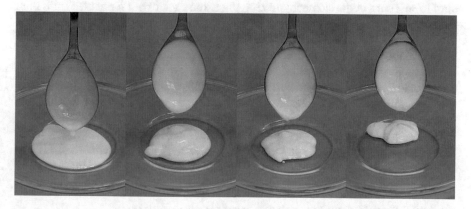

Yogurt-like fermented milk products vary in both flavor and consistency. (Wikimedia Commons User Nillerdk, taken March 19 2009)

LAB fermentation is characterized by the conversion of carbohydrates to lactic acid, which lowers the pH of the product. The rapid acidification by LAB inhibits growth of microorganisms that lead to spoilage and can even prevent the proliferation of some pathogens. Certain strains of LAB, such as *Lactobacillus plantarum* and *Lactobacillus coryniformis*, have been regarded for their antifungal properties, specifically in the ability to inhibit the growth of *Penicillium expansum*, *Penicillium commune*, *Fusarium sporotrichioides* and the yeast *Rhodotorula mucilaginosa* which are related with food spoilage and harmful mold in fermented milk (Magnusson et al., 2003; Tulini et al., 2016). Particularly harmful pathogenic strains of *Escherichia coli* and *Salmonella enteritidis* found in milk were also inhibited by a strain of the LAB *Lactococcus lactic* due to its fast acid production and ability to quickly lower pH (Mufandaedza et al., 2006). Recent developments in pasteurization technologies have further enhanced the safety and extended the shelf life of fresh and fermented milk products. These methods involve UHT (ultra-high temperature) pasteurization and the application of pulsed electric fields, ultrasound, and ultraviolet light to milk (Datta & Tomasula, 2015). LAB strains continue to be studied for their beneficial ability to preserve milk.

The breakdown of proteins by LAB in milk results in the release of bioactive compounds and free amino acids, with application to immunostimulating activity and health promoting properties. The hydrolysis of caseins by LAB has been noted for its peptide release related to antihypertension, and antimicrobial activity, while whey hydrolysis has been associated with other bioactive molecules related to cholesterol-lowering and immunomodulating activity (Meisel, 2005; Pessione & Cirrincione, 2016; Tellez et al., 2010). LAB protein degradation in fermented milk products have a major impact on not only the nutritional value of the product, but also the matrix structure, functional characteristics, and especially flavor compounds (Li et al., 2019, 3699). These fermentation organisms can even convert hard curd to soft curd in the stomach; making digestion easier with fermented milk than with liquid milk. This process also allows fermented milk proteins to be more easily accessible, and thus more useful, for children, older people, and those with stomach ulcers. While the proteins in milk are generally considered to be of "excellent biological quality" and both caseins and whey proteins are well endowed with essential amino acids, the protein content of fermented milk is often elevated by concentrations or addition of skim milk solids, allowing for an even more attractive source of protein than liquid milk (Table 7.1) (Khedkar et al., 2016).

A similar relationship occurs with vitamins and minerals (Table 7.2). Milk products are a particularly great source of vitamins, including riboflavin, vitamins B6, B12, A, D, K and E. LAB have been studied for their ability to synthesize some

Table 7.2 Effect of fermentation on vitamin content of milk (mg/100 g)

Vitamins	Whole milk	Buttermilk	Sour cream	Yogurt	Cottage cheese
Thiamin	30	34	35	44	21
Riboflavin	170	154	149	214	165
Niacin	100	58	67	114	128
Pantothenic acid	300	275	360	591	215
Vitamin B_6	40	34	16	49	68
Folacin	6	Traces	11	11	12
Vitamin B_{12}	0.04	0.22	0.30	0.56	0.63

Khedkar, C. D., Khedkar, G. D., Chavan, N. V. and Kalyankar, S. D. (2003). Fermented milks: Dietary importance. In: Encyclopaedia of Food Science and Nutrition (2nd ed.). London: Elsevier

water-soluble vitamins, especially certain B vitamins such as folate, riboflavin, and vitamin B12 (Leblanc et al., 2011; Pacheco Da Silva et al., 2016; Zironi et al., 2014). Fat-soluble vitamins such as vitamin K has also been shown to increase in fermented milk products, which has importance in promoting bone health and preventing cardiovascular disease (Melini et al., 2019; Walther et al., 2013). Minerals in fermented milk products such as calcium, phosphate, zinc and magnesium have been observed for their increased bioavailability (Bergillos-Meca et al., 2015; De La Fuente et al., 2003). Improved calcium absorption from fermented milk products such as yogurt has been especially contentious but many studies agree that fermented milk products are a rich source of calcium for lactose intolerant individuals and may improve calcium uptake (He et al., 2005; Hodges et al., 2019, 8).

7.3 Solving "The Milk Problem"

Dairy milk has been embroiled in debates of not only health but also safety for centuries. The components of milk (carbohydrates, fats, proteins, and water) provide an ideal site for the growth of harmful pathogens like *Salmonella, Escherichia coli, Listeria monocytogenes, Mycobacterium tuberculosis, and Brucella* (Valenze, 2015,1178–1179). In the mid-nineteenth century, the early years of dairy industrialization, poor sanitation during production and transportation of milk to growing cities like London and New York proved deadly. "Distillery slop dairies," so named because of the leftover slop from local distilleries and breweries fed to the cows, were characterized by sick animals, lack of ventilation, and heaps of waste (Velten, 2010, 59–60) The "whiskey milk" produced by these infected animals was often cut with contaminated water or plaster of Paris to stretch production. Detailed reports of poor production conditions, including a *New York Times* article estimating that swill milk had caused the death of nearly 10,000 infants in New York, led to calls for reform in the US (Lytton, 2019, 27). During this period, the mysterious "white elixir" earned a new moniker: "white poison" (Velten, 2010, 66).

Pasteur's nineteenth century efforts to understand and control invisible microorganisms led to a host of staggering theoretical and practice uses, ranging from the first vaccines to the sanitation process now known as *pasteurization*. Developed in 1863 as a technique to preserve wine (and ultimately save this important French from collapse), the early iterations of pasteurization involved a relatively simple process of heating perishable liquids to 120–140 ° F to kill off harmful bacteria. Still, it did not become widespread in the dairy industry for several decades. Despite conflict between consumers and producers, local and federal governments, and private and public entities (Lytton, 2019, 53–54), Chicago became the first US city to implement legislation requiring the pasteurization of milk in 1908, followed shortly thereafter by New York City in 1910 and other major cities throughout the decade (Czaplicki, 2007, 411–433). These laws were followed by a cascade of subsequent regulations, heavily lobbied by interest groups, monitored by the newly-established

Food and Drug Association, aimed at ensuring safe milk products at prices supported by the market. The science and policy of solving "the Milk Problem" would lay the foundation for the United States' food safety infrastructure, including government agencies, research institutions, and citizen initiatives (Lytton, 2019, 41).

Recent developments in pasteurization technologies have further enhanced the safety and extended the shelf life of fresh and fermented milk products. These methods involve UHT (ultra-high temperature) pasteurization and the application of pulsed electric fields, ultrasound, and ultraviolet light to milk (Datta & Tomasula, 2015), among others. Still, the issue of post-pasteurization contamination (PPC) remains a problem in the United States, with 50% of fluid milk showing evidence of PPC (Martin et al., 2018, 861). For this reason, the safety of pasteurized dairy milk continues to depend on system-level considerations including transportation and storage.

7.4 Health Benefits on a Grander Scale

In 2008, scientists working for Danisco, a biotech company that makes yogurt, were researching ways to stabilize the starter of its yogurt culture and came across what many already believe may be the greatest discovery of the twenty-first century, the Clustered Regularly Interspaced Short Palindromic Repeats (CRISPR). CRISPR has been acknowledged as a scientific breakthrough in the identification of bacteria that is resistant to infections by bacteriophages (Daniells, 2007) and has dramatic implications for the study of the human genome and the potential to cure genetic diseases with a precise gene-editing technique. Milk may be the basis for the creation of the Milky Way in myths and folklore but fermented milk, long regarded as an elixir of life, may be a basis for deepening the understanding of the human body and the ability to "cure" previously incurable diseases and extend healthy life.

7.5 Social and Environmental Questions in the Yogurt Industry

Though an Armenian immigrant to the US named Sarkis Colombosian began selling yogurt out of his small creamery in Andover, Massachusetts in 1929 (Adams, 2021), yogurt did not gain mainstream popularity in the US until the counterculture movement of the 1960s and 1970s. A derivative of milk, which over several decades had been deemed "nature's perfect food" (Dupuis, 2002, 3–16), yogurt was recast in the American imaginary as an elitist health food, detached from all cultural context, and quickly became the fastest growing segment of the dairy industry. In fact, yogurt sales saw a 200% increase in the 70s and 80s (Gurel, 2016, 69).

FAGE, a Greek company, introduced strained yogurt to American supermarkets in 1998, initiating the association of this previously unfamiliar, thick, tart yogurt with Greece, despite the fact that strained yogurt is popular in many parts of the Mediterranean and Middle East. When Hamdi Ulukaya, a Turkish immigrant to the US, founded Chobani in 2005 in the post-9/11 context of widespread Islamophobia, he opted to maintain this association and market his product as "Greek" (Gurel, 2016, 74). The strategy was successful and Ulukaya's competitors followed suit one after another with brands like Dannon's Oikos, Yoplait's Greek 100, and Greek Gods.

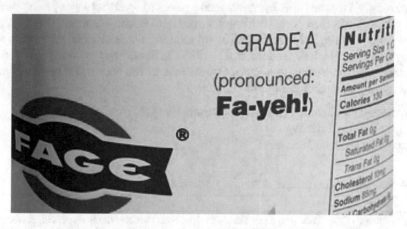

Fage, a Greek company, was the first to introduce strained yogurt to US consumers on a large scale. (Wikimedia Commons Author Yoshi Canopus taken 9, September 2015)

As fad diets in the United States shifted from low fat in the 1980s to low carb in the 1990s (La Berge, 2008, 168), yogurt companies maintained their product's importance as a health food by fastidiously targeting women dieters. By removing both fat and sugar from yogurt products and marketing them as "indulgences," yogurt became associated not only with health but also thin, well-regulated female bodies. Touting 0% fat, no added sugar, beneficial probiotics, and flat tummies in its commercials, Danone's Activia brand exemplifies the corporate gendering of yogurt consumption. By the mid-2000s, brands of Greek yogurt sought to expand their consumer base by targeting men, who previously made up only one third of the market (Contois, 2019). "Brogurt" advertisements highlighted high protein content, NFL affiliations, dark packaging, larger portions, and ribbed containers meant to simulate the appearance of six-pack abs (Contois, 2020, 77).

Contemporary diets high in animal protein among consumers in wealthy, industrialized countries have been linked to a variety of environmental problems, including climate altering emissions (von der Pahlen, 2018, 34) and excessive water use (Hoekstra & Chapagain, 2007, 40). In addition to this, the massive volume of acid whey produced by industrial yogurt companies has proven a difficult challenge for dairy industry professionals and policymakers to manage. In 2015 alone, strained yogurt production in the US resulted in nearly 1.5 million tons of acid whey (Erickson, 2017), and spills of the byproduct have reportedly killed tens of thousands of fish across the country by acidifying waterways and robbing streams and rivers of oxygen (Elliott, 2021). As a result, dairy scientists, corporations, and entrepreneurs have worked to turn this environmental threat into an economic opportunity. Solutions to the acid whey problem range from converting it to biofuel through anaerobic digestion to repurposing residual proteins for baby food (Elliott, 2021). Additionally, General Mills has developed a patent to revert acid whey into "sweet" whey, which can then be used in protein powder (Rocha-Mendoza, 2021, 1264). Others are exploring the market viability of fermented milk drinks using excess acid whey as a base (Rocha-Mendoza, 2021, 1265). In these ways, with the aid of modern technology, this new iteration of "white poison" has once again been reconfigured as a highly-regarded superfood (Table 7.3).

"My Mother's Tarator" (Bulgarian Yogurt Soup)
Recipe by Elitsa Stoyneva
Adapted by Danielle Jacques

Table 7.3 Fermentation induced changes in milk constituents

Constituents	Changes
Milk proteins (3–4.5%)	Coagulated into a smooth curd with casein particles finely dispersed. Partially peptonized (0.1–0.7%) and utilized for microbial growth, resulting in the buildup of microbial cell proteins, increase in nonprotein nitrogen, and release of peptides and amino acids
Lactose (4.5–5%)	Partially utilized (1–2%) by starter bacteria producing mainly lactic acid (0.6–2%), volatile acids, flavor compounds, and CO_2 may also be formed by heterofermentative types. Alcohol and CO_2 may be produced by lactose-fermenting yeasts
Milk fat (3.5–7%)	Fermentation leads to partial digestion of lipids
Mineral matter (0.7–0.8%)	No direct appreciable change
Vitamins	No change in fat-soluble vitamins A, D, E, and K. Slight decrease in B-complex vitamins depending on the strains used

Khedkar, C. D., Khedkar, G. D., Chavan, N. V. and Kalyankar, S. D. (2003). Fermented milks: Dietary importance. In: Encyclopaedia of Food Science and Nutrition (2nd ed.). London: Elsevier

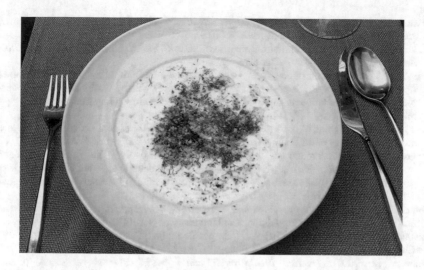

Photo of tarator taken by author (Jacques) in Varna, Bulgaria

Ingredients:

> 1 Large cucumber (200–350 g)
> 400 g Bulgarian Yogurt (plain, whole milk, unstrained)
> 1 tbsp dried dill or one small bunch of fresh dill
> 2 cloves of garlic
> 150 ml of water
> 1 1/2 tsp. of salt
> 2 tbsp sunflower oil (can substitute olive oil)
> 30 g walnuts, chopped

Directions:

1. Peel and cut cucumber into small cubes (the size of a small dice) and place in a bowl. Finely crush garlic cloves and add to the bowl. Add salt and mix gently. Let sit for 4–5 minutes.
2. In a large bowl, stir yogurt until smooth.
3. Add water to the yogurt. Mix well. Add dill and salted cucumber-garlic mixture.
4. Add oil and finely chopped walnuts. Garnish with extra dill.
5. Serve cold.

References

Abarca, M. E. (2013). Culinary encounters in Latino/a literature (Part III: Traditions). In S. Bost & F. R. Aparicio (Eds.), *The Routledge companion to Latino/a literature* (pp. 251–260). Routledge, Taylor & Francis Group.

Adams, T. (2021). *Andover's role in the history of yogurt*. [Online] Andover Townsman. Available at: https://www.andovertownsman.com/news/townspeople/andovers-role-in-the-history-of-yogurt/article_0931ed7f-42c8-5757-a0b5-7767c9001df8.html. Accessed 27 May 2021.

Aryana, K. J., & Olson, D. W. (2017). A 100-year review: Yogurt and other cultured dairy products. *Journal of Dairy Science, 100*(12), 9987–10013.

Barker, J. S. F. (2014). Water Buffalo: Domestication. In C. Smith (Ed.), *Encyclopedia of Global Archaeology* (pp. 7694–7697). Springer.

Bergillos-Meca, T., Cabrera-Vique, C., Artacho, R., Moreno-Montoro, M., Navarro-Alarcón, M., Olalla, M., Giménez, R., Seiquer, I., & Ruiz-López, M. D. (2015). Does Lactobacillus plantarum or ultrafiltration process improve Ca, Mg, Zn and P bioavailability from fermented goats' milk? *Food Chemistry, 187*, 314–321.

Chen, S., Lin, B.-Z., Baig, M., Mitra, B., Lopes, R. J., Santos, A. M., et al. (2010). Zebu cattle are an exclusive legacy of the South Asia Neolithic. *Molecular Biology and Evolution, 27*(1), 1–6.

Contois, E. (2019). 'Protein in the macronutrient imaginary: The case of "Brogurt" marketing.' *H-Nutrition | H-Net* [Online]. Available at: https://networks.h-net.org/node/134048/discussions/4443764/protein-macronutrient-imaginary-case-%E2%80%9Cbrogurt%E2%80%9D. Accessed 2020 Aug 24.

Contois, E. J. H. (2020). *Diners, dudes, and diets: How gender and power collide in food media and culture* (p. 77). Illustrated edition. The University of North Carolina Press.

Czaplicki, A. (2007). "Pure milk is better than purified milk": Pasteurization and milk purity in Chicago, 1908–1916. *Social Science History, 31*(3), 411–433.

Daniells, S. (2007). *Danisco breakthrough could boost cultures' resistance.* [Online] foodnavigator-usa.com. Available at: https://www.foodnavigator-usa.com/Article/2007/03/23/Danisco-breakthrough-could-boost-cultures-resistance?utm_source=copyright&utm_medium=OnSite&utm_campaign=copyright. Accessed 31 May 2021.

Datta, N., & Tomasula, P. M. (2015). *Emerging dairy processing technologies: Opportunities for the dairy industry [Internet].* John Wiley & Sons, Incorporated.

De La Fuente, M. A., Montes, F., Guerrero, G., & Juárez, M. (2003). Total and soluble contents of calcium, magnesium, phosphorus and zinc in yoghurts. *Food Chemistry, 80*, 573–578.

Dupuis, E. M. (2002). *Nature's perfect food: How milk became America's drink* (pp. 3–16). NYU Press, New York University Press.

Elliott, J. (2021) Whey too much: Greek yogurt's dark side. [Online] Modern Farmer. Available at: https://modernfarmer.com/2013/05/whey-too-much-greek-yogurts-dark-side/#:~:text=The%20resulting%20whey%20is%20roughly,very%20small%20amount%20of%20proteins. Accessed 16 Aug 2021.

Erickson, B. (2017). 'Acid whey: Is the waste product an untapped goldmine?' Chemical & Engineering News. Available at: https://cen.acs.org/articles/95/i6/Acid-whey-waste-product-untapped.html. Accessed 16 Aug 2021.

Evershed, R. P., Payne, S., Sherratt, A. G., Copley, M. S., Coolidge, J., Urem-Kotsu, D., et al. (2008). Earliest date for milk use in the Near East and southeastern Europe linked to cattle herding. *Nature, 455*(7212), 528–531.

Fisberg, M., & Machado, R. (2015). History of yogurt and current patterns of consumption. *Nutrition Reviews, 73*, 4–7.

Gasbarrini, G., Bonvicini, F., & Gramenzi, A. (2016). Probiotics history. *Journal of Clinical Gastroenterology, 50*, S116–S119.

Geissler, C., & Powers, H. (2010). *Human nutrition* (12th ed., p. 34). Churchill Livingstone.

Gurel, P. (2016). Live and active cultures: Gender, ethnicity, and "Greek" yogurt in America. *Gastronomica, 16*(4), 66–77.

Haug, A., Høstmark, A. T., & Harstad, O. M. (2007). Bovine milk in human nutrition – A review. *Lipids in Health and Disease, 6*, 25.

He, M., Yang, Y. X., Han, H., Men, J. H., Bian, L. H., & Wang, G. D. (2005). Effects of yogurt supplementation on the growth of preschool children in Beijing suburbs. *Biomedical and Environmental Sciences, 18*, 192–197.

Hodges, J., Cao, S., Cladis, D., & Weaver, C. (2019). Lactose intolerance and bone health: The challenge of ensuring adequate calcium intake. *Nutrients, 11*, 1–17.

Hoekstra, A. Y., & Chapagain, A. K. (2007). Water footprints of nations: Water use by people as a function of their consumption pattern. *Water Resources Management, 21,* 35–48.

Itan, Y., Powell, A., Beaumont, M. A., Burger, J., & Thomas, M. G. (2009). The Origins of Lactase Persistence in Europe. *PLoS Computational Biology, 5*(8), 1–13.

Ji-Young Park, S. (2011). Algeria. In K. Albala (Ed.), *Food Cultures of the World Encyclopedia. – African and Middle East* (Vol. 1). ABC-CLIO, LLC. 22.

Khedkar, C. D., Kalyankar, S. D., & Deosarkar, S. S. (2016). Fermented foods: Fermented milks. In B. Caballero, P. Finglas, & F. Toldrá (Eds.), *The Encyclopedia of Food and Health* (Vol. 2, pp. 661–667). Academic.

Kindairy. (2021). *KIN yogurt*. [Online] Available at: https://www.kindairy.com/en/kin-yogurt. Accessed 27 May 2021.

Kindstedt, P. (2012). *Cheese and culture: A history of cheese and its place in western civilization* (p. 10). Chelsea Green Pub.

Laudan, R. (2015). *Cuisine and empire: Cooking in world history* (p. 28). University of California.

Leblanc, J. G., Laiño, J. E., Del Valle, M. J., Vannini, V., Van Sinderen, D., Taranto, M. P., De Valdez, G. F., De Giori, G. S., & Sesma, F. (2011). B-Group vitamin production by lactic acid bacteria – Current knowledge and potential applications. *Journal of Applied Microbiology, 111,* 1297–1309.

Leroy, F., & De Vuyst, L. (2004). Lactic acid bacteria as functional starter cultures for the food fermentation industry. *Trends in Food Science and Technology, 15,* 67–78.

Li, S., Tang, S., He, Q., Hu, J., & Zheng, J. (2019). Changes in proteolysis in fermented milk produced by Streptococcus thermophilus in co-culture with Lactobacillus plantarum or Bifidobacterium animalis subsp. lactis during refrigerated storage. *Molecules, 24,* 3699.

Lytton, T. D. (2019). *Outbreak: Foodborne illness and the struggle for food safety*. The University of Chicago Press.

Magnusson, J., Ström, K., Roos, S., Sjögren, J., & Schnürer, J. (2003). Broad and complex antifungal activity among environmental isolates of lactic acid bacteria. *FEMS Microbiology Letters, 219,* 129–135.

Martin, N. H., Boor, K. J., & Wiedmann, M. (2018). Symposium review: Effect of post-pasteurization contamination on fluid milk quality. *Journal of Dairy Science, 101*(1), 861–870.

Meiji.com. (2021). *Meiji Co., Ltd. | Meiji Holdings Co., Ltd.* [Online] Available at: https://www.meiji.com/global/about-us/corporate-profile/meiji/business-categories/international/. Accessed 27 May 2021.

Meisel, H. (2005). Biochemical properties of peptides encrypted in bovine milk proteins. *Current Medicinal Chemistry, 12,* 1905–1919.

Melini, F., Melini, V., Luziatelli, F., Ficca, A. G., & Ruzzi, M. (2019). Health-promoting components in fermented foods: An up-to-date systematic review. *Nutrients, 11,* 1189.

Mlekuž, D. (2015). Archaeological culture, please meet yoghurt culture: Towards a relational archaeology of milk. *Documenta Praehistorica, 42,* 275–288.

Mudgal, S., & Prajapati, J. (2017). Chapter 20 – Dahi: An Indian naturally fermented yogurt. In R. C. Chandan, A. Gandhi, & N. P. Shah (Eds.), *Yogurt in health and disease prevention* (pp. 353–369). Academic.

Mufandaedza, J., Viljoen, B. C., Feresu, S. B., & Gadaga, T. H. (2006). Antimicrobial properties of lactic acid bacteria and yeast-lab cultures isolated from traditional fermented milk against pathogenic Escherichia Coli and Salmonella Enteritidis strains. *International Journal of Food Microbiology, 108,* 147–152.

Ozen, M., & Dinleyici, E. (2015). The history of probiotics: The untold story. *Beneficial Microbes, 6,* 1–7.

Pacheco Da Silva, F. F., Biscola, V., Leblanc, J. G., De Melo, G., & Franco, B. D. (2016). Effect of indigenous lactic acid bacteria isolated from goat milk and cheeses on folate and riboflavin content of fermented goat milk. *LWT - Food Science and Technology, 71,* 155–161.

Pessione, E., & Cirrincione, S. (2016). Bioactive molecules released in food by lactic acid bacteria: Encrypted peptides and biogenic amines. *Frontiers in Microbiology, 7.*

Sen, C. T. (2015). *Feasts and fasts: A history of food in India* (p. 211). Reaktion Books, Limited.

Stoilova, E. (2015). The bulgarianization of yoghurt: Connecting home, taste, and authenticity. *Food & Foodways, 23*(1–2), 14–35.

Tellez, A., Corredig, M., Brovko, L. Y., & Griffiths, M. W. (2010). Characterization of immune-active peptides obtained from milk fermented by Lactobacillus Helveticus. *The Journal of Dairy Research, 77,* 129–136.

Tulini, F. L., Hymery, N., Haertlé, T., Le Blay, G., & De Martinis, E. C. (2016). Screening for anti-microbial and proteolytic activities of lactic acid bacteria isolated from cow, buffalo and goat milk and cheeses marketed in the southeast region of Brazil. *The Journal of Dairy Research, 83,* 115–124.

Turnbull, A. (2012). Kumis/Airag. In J. Deutsch & N. Murakhver (Eds.), *They eat that?: A cultural Encyclopedia of weird and exotic food from around the world.* ABC-CLIO, LLC. 128.

Valenze, D. (2011). *Milk: A local and global history* (pp. 5–50). Yale University Press.

Valenze, D. (2015). Raw milk and pasteurization. *The SAGE Encyclopedia of Food Issues,* 1178–1181.

Velten, H. (2010). *Milk a global history.* Reaktion Books.

von der Pahlen, C. T. (2018). Climate change and sustainable and healthy diets. In B. Burlingame & S. Dernini (Eds.), *Sustainable diets: Linking nutrition and food systems.* CAB International.

Walther, B., Karl, J. P., Booth, S. L., & Boyaval, P. (2013). Menaquinones, bacteria, and the food supply: The relevance of dairy and fermented food products to vitamin K requirements. *Advances In Nutrition (Bethesda, Md), 4,* 463–473.

Wiley, A. S. (2014). *Cultures of milk: The biology and meaning of dairy products in the United States and India* (p. 58). Harvard University Press.

World food company – Danone. (2021). Living Heritage. [Online] Available at: https://www.danone.com/about-danone/ourhistory.html. Accessed 27 May 2021.

Wouters, J. T. M., Ayad, E. H. E., Hugenholtz, J., & Smit, G. (2002). Microbes from raw milk for fermented dairy products. *International Dairy Journal, 12,* 91–109.

Yotova, M. (2018). Ethnographic Heritage as a branding strategy: A case study of yogurt in Bulgaria and Japan. *Global Economic Review, 47*(1), 47–62.

Zironi, E., Gazzotti, T., Barbarossa, A., Farabegoli, F., Serraino, A., & Pagliuca, G. (2014). Determination of vitamin B(12) in dairy products by ultra performance liquid chromatography-tandem mass spectrometry. *Italian Journal of Food Safety, 3,* 4513.

Chapter 8
Ginger

Amy Kousch

8.1 Cultural History

Ginger (*Zingeber officinale*) is a perennial, flowering plant of the Zingeberaceae family, which includes over 50 genera and around 1400 named species (Buhner, 2013; Nair, 2019). The genus *Zingeber* includes the commonly cultivated culinary and medicinal plant, *Zingeber officinale. Zingeber officinale* has been used as a source of medicine and food in China and India for over 4000 years (Akbar, 2020). The word Zingeber (Latin) has etymological roots in Tamil (South India) and translates to "ginger rhizome" (Nair, 2013, p. 249). The precise geographic origin of ginger is unknown, but it is believed to have evolved in Southeast Asia. Ginger's rhizome (a modified stem) is the well-recognized plant part cultivated for therapeutic and culinary use.

8.2 Traditional Chinese Medicine

In traditional Chinese medicine (TCM), ginger is used to treat many illnesses. Chinese practitioners use fresh ginger rhizome (*Sheng jiang*) or the mature, dried rhizome (*Gan Jiang*) as separately unique applications of medicine (Akbar, 2020; Nair, 2019). TCM describes *Shen jiang* as having warm and acrid properties, a pungent taste, and a warm nature (Akbar, 2020; Nair, 2019). *Sheng jiang* is used to treat the following ailments: nausea, vomiting, stagnated Qi energy, vertigo, pregnancy induced nausea and vomiting, early onset of viral infections, headaches, nasal congestion, coughs, and other respiratory issues (Akbar, 2020; Nair, 2019). TCM

A. Kousch (✉)
Berchta Botanicals, Fort Collins, CO, USA
e-mail: info@berchtabotanicals.com

values *Sheng jiang* for its anti-inflammatory, antitussive, and detoxicant properties (Akbar, 2020; Nair, 2019). *Gan Jiang* is primarily used to treat abdominal pain, diarrhea, and other digestive issues and is categorized as having hot properties and a pungent taste (Akbar, 2020; Nair, 2019).

8.3 Ayurvedic Medicine

Ginger is one of oldest healing herbs found in Ayurvedic texts. It is used to stimulate warmth, circulation, digestion, and energy and is described as acrid and digestive (Buhner, 2013). Ginger has many names in ancient Ayurvedic texts. It is often called *'Mahaoushadha'* or, the great cure (Nair, 2013 p. 249). In Ayurvedic medicine, ginger is used as an anti-inflammatory and antiedematous agent (Nair, 2019). It used to assist with asthmatic conditions, bronchial issues, and for cleansing the throat (Buhner, 2013; Mao et al., 2019). Ginger is used in cough remedies, to strengthen the memory, and as a diuretic (Buhner, 2013; Mao et al., 2019). This is not an exhaustive list of ginger's prominence and presence in Ayurvedic healing. Ginger plays an integral role in Ayurvedic treatments.

8.4 Traditional Western Medicine

Ginger is primarily used in traditional western medicine (TWM) to alleviate digestive issues, as an anti-inflammatory, and to aid with nausea and vomiting. Ginger's use as an antiemetic and antinausea treatment is well known and has been extensively studied (Nair, 2019). Ginger is used to treat motion sickness, post-operation nausea (N) and vomiting (V), pregnancy induced N and V, headaches and migraine associated N and V and any N and V arising as side effects of illnesses, medications, or external factors (Akbar, 2020; Buhner, 2013; Nair, 2019).

8.5 Ginger in Nutrition and Health Research

Ginger has been used as a healing herb for thousands of years. Decades of studies show that ginger contains anti-inflammatory, chemo preventative, antiatherogenic, blood-pressure lowering, hypoglycemic, antibacterial, antiviral, anti-fungal, anti-infective, cardioprotective and antimicrobial, antispasmodic, antiatherosclerotic, analgesic, antipyretic, diaphoretic, carminative, and antioxidant properties (Grzanna et al., 2005; Nair, 2019; Odle, 2014; Rupasinghe & Gunathilake, 2015; Sharifi-Rad et al., 2017). According to Mao et al. (2019 p. 185), ginger is *"rich in various chemical constituents, including phenolic compounds, terpenes, polysaccharides, lipids, organic acids, and raw fibers.*" Ginger is rich in Vitamin A, Vitamin C, manganese, sodium, chlorine, and iron. Chemical analyses of ginger rhizomes demonstrate the following nutritional profile: 8.6% protein, 6.4% fat, and 5.9% fiber (Attokaran, 2017; Nair, 2019; Rupasinghe & Gunathilake, 2015).

8.6 Plant Constituents

Over 400 constituents have been identified in ginger rhizomes (Buhner, 2013; Grzanna et al., 2005). These include: gingerol, shogaol, zingiberene, phellandrene, borneol, zerumbone, 3-dihydroshogoal, dihydroparadol and more. Many of the studied pharmacological properties of ginger have been traced, largely, to gingerol, shogaol, and paradol compounds (Butt & Sultan, 2011; Grzanna et al., 2005; Mao et al., 2019; Nair, 2019; Rupasinghe & Gunathilake, 2015; Sharifi-Rad et al., 2017).

8.7 Gingerols and Anti-inflammatory Action

Gingerols refer to the chains of molecules, found in ginger, of various lengths, with potent pharmacological value (Butt & Sultan, 2011; Grzanna et al., 2005; Mao et al., 2019; Nair, 2019; Rupasinghe & Gunathilake, 2015; Sang, 2020; Sharifi-Rad et al., 2017). The most abundant of gingerols is 6-gingerol. Gingerol is most plentiful in the fresh rhizome of ginger and is converted to shogoal during ginger's post-harvest drying process (Grzanna et al., 2005; Nair, 2019; Rupasinghe & Gunathilake, 2015; Sharifi-Rad et al., 2017). Gingerol's anti-inflammatory action is achieved through the inhibition of the biosynthesis of prostaglandins (PGs), cyclooxygenase 1 and 2 (COX-1 and COX-2), and lipoxygenase (LOX) pathways (Grzanna et al., 2005; Nair, 2019; Rupasinghe & Gunathilake, 2015; Sang, 2020; Sharifi-Rad et al., 2017). Arachidonic acid metabolism functions as a precursor to both COX and LOX pathways which result in the presence both PG and Leukotrienes (LT). PG and LT activate cellular inflammatory responses. Gingerol inhibits PG and LT synthesis by blocking COX and LOX metabolism of arachidonic acid (Grzanna et al., 2005, Nair, 2019, Rupasinghe & Gunathilake, 2015, Sharifi-Rad et al., 2017). Additionally, ginger has been shown to block cytokine activation at cellular sites (Grzanna et al., 2005; Nair, 2019; Rupasinghe & Gunathilake, 2015; Sharifi-Rad et al., 2017).

8.8 Arthritic Conditions

Numerous studies over many years indicate the use of ginger to alleviate arthritic pain and swelling due to its anti-inflammatory properties. Bliddal et al. (2000) performed a placebo-controlled study examining the potency of ginger as compared to ibuprofen for arthritic conditions which demonstrated positive results for ginger's effectiveness as a pain reducer (cited in Nair, 2019). Altman and Marcussen (cited in Akbar, 2020) carried out a 6-month double blind placebo study with 29 patients with results pointing to pain reduction as a result of ginger use. In Srivastava and Mustafa's 1989 study (cited in Nair, 2019), 75% of patients receiving ginger reported a reduction in arthritic related pain and inflammation. Again, 6-gingerol blocks inflammatory responses at the cellular level and greatly decreases arthritic pain as a result.

8.9   Neurodegenerative Disease

As a defensive response to external stress, microglial cells will become inflamed. This inflammatory response is designed to allow for tissue repair, however, chronically activated microglial cells lead to the pronounced neuron loss that is observed in neurodegenerative diseases (Azam, 2014; Grzanna et al., 2005). Ginger has been studied to block the process leading up to inflammatory responses in microglial cells. The phenyl rings and hydroxy rings specific to ginger compounds are responsible for targeting and regulating cellular pathways. Studies performed on brain matter in patients with Parkinson's disease, dementia, and Alzheimer's disease demonstrate that inflammation is a principle driver of central nervous system degeneration (Grzanna et al., 2005).

8.10   Other Health Benefits

Fresh ginger has been used as an antiviral medicine for thousands of years (Buhner, 2013). It has been studied to be effective against "colds, influenza, hepatitis, herpes, yellow fever, measles, chicken pox and enterovirus" (Buhner, 2013, p.172). Gingerol acts as an inhibitory agent and a virucidal. Buhner states, "It blocks the attachments of viruses to cells, inhibits hemagglutinin, viral proteases, neuramindase and promotes antiviral macrophage activity" (Buhner, 2013, p.172). Ginger is effective against the growth of bacteria, including: *Listeria spp., Haemophilus influenza* and *Streptococcus viridans* (Buhner, 2013). The essential oil of ginger exhibits antimicrobial activity against all Gram positive and Gram negative tested bacteria as well as against *Salmonella tyhphimurium, Escherichia coli* and *Shigella dysenteriae*, among many other microbial agents (Akbar, 2020; Nair, 2019; Rupasinghe & Gunathilake, 2015).

8.11 Ginger

A Survey of Botany, Biology, and Chemistry Ginger (*Zingeber officinale*) is a member of the Zingiberacaea family and, along with Galangal, Turmeric, and Cardamom, is a member of the genus Zingeber. Many of the Zingeber species demonstrate similar healing actions. Plants in this family share alternative and distichous leaves with a sheathed base and lance shape (Babu & Ravindran, 2004). The flowers in this genus are bisexual and exhibit zygomorphic traits. Flower bracts are often supported on a raceme. In 1807, botanist William Roscoe described ginger in the Botanic Garden of Livermore and thus named ginger, *Zingeber officinale* Roscoe (Babu & Ravindran, 2004). *Zingeber officinale* Roscoe is therefore sometimes used as a moniker for this commonly used medicinal and culinary plant (Nair, 2013; Parthasarathy et al., 2011).

Ginger grows to about two to three feet high on an erect cane-like stem and has sheathing, lance shaped leaves and irregular yellowish-green to white flowers (Buhner, 2013). As a commodity crop, ginger is grown as an annual and is commercially cultivated for its rhizome (underground stem). The rhizome presents as a "thick, laterally compressed, and palmately branched modified storage organ with light, yellow flesh inside and exterior scales" (Parthasarathy et al., 2011, p. 281). The first developed rhizome is referred to as the mother rhizome. Parthasarathy et al. describes the subsequent growth of tillers and fingers, "The mother rhizome branches on either side and grow out to become the primary tillers, the base of which will enlarge and become the primary fingers. The buds on these primary fingers will develop into secondary tillers and their bases into secondary fingers. The buds on the secondary fingers in turn can develop into tertiary tillers and tertiary fingers" (p. 282).

Ginger has both fibrous and fleshy roots which extend from the base of sprouted rhizomes. The main function of the fibrous roots is to absorb water and nutrients from the rhizosphere. The fleshy roots provide support as well as engage in minor nutrient uptake (Sharifi-Rad et al., 2017).

Previously, this chapter discussed ginger's pharmacological benefits as a medicinal plant. The medicinal properties of ginger are largely attributed to its gingerols and shogoals. Gingerols are phenolic compounds which are formed from hexonate, malonate and phenylalanine (Grzanna et al., 2005). Constituents of ginger's volatile oil include: sesquiterpenes, camphene, curcumin, terpineol, terpenes, limonene, linalool, alpha-zingerberence and beta-sesquiphellandrene (Grzanna et al., 2005). Gingerol is a hydroxymethoxyphenol compound (HAPC). HAPC contribute to the inhibition of PG synthesis –thereby preventing inflammation (Grzanna et al., 2005).

Figure 8.1 below illustrates major botanical features of the ginger plant.

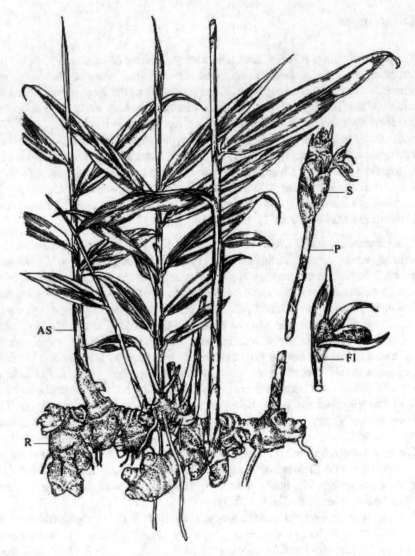

Fig. 8.1 Drawing of ginger plant outlining the shoots, inflorescence, and flower. AS: Aerial shoot, R: Rhizome, Fl: Flower, P: Peduncle (scape), S: Spike (Source: Babu & Ravindran, 2004, p.19)

8.12 Ginger Cultivation

Sustainability and Agricultural Issues Ginger has been cultivated as food and medicine crop for around 4000 years in Asia (Buhner, 2013). It is believed to have originated in tropical Southeast Asia (Parthasarathy et al., 2011). The plant is a perennial that thrives in warm, humid climates with rich soil, abundant water, and indirect sunlight (Buhner, 2013).

India (30% of world production) and China (20% of world production) account for half of the word's ginger production (Nair, 2013). Other significant ginger producing countries include: Thailand, Brazil, Taiwan, Nigeria, and Indonesia (Nair, 2013). Globally, there are markets for three 'types' of ginger: fresh ginger, preserved fresh ginger, and dried ginger (Nair, 2013). As a matter of international trade, the global ginger market is orchestrated by firms and individual brokers (Nair, 2013).

Ginger is grown in a wide range of soil types – differences in geographically unique soil types impact, as a consequence, the growth ouput, days to maturity, and constituent concentrations of varied ginger ecotypes (Parthasarathy et al., 2011; Sharifi-Rad et al., 2017). Ginger prefers a soil pH in the 6.0–6.5 range and generally thrives in loamy soils with a high humus content. Although ginger can tolerate a spectrum of sandy loam to loamy clay soils, Whiley (1974) and Cho et al. (1987) reported that ginger yields will decrease when growing in heavy clay or soils with exceptionally low PH (cited in Parthasarathy et al., 2011). Broadly speaking, ginger's life cycle as a cultivated crop is determined by geographic location, climate, and soil type. Ginger rhizomes are usually planted between February and June depending on the country. Rhizomes are planted as early as frost-free dates and other farming factors permit to allow the plant to develop a stable root and stem system so that the crop can withstand heavy, soaking rains (Parthasarathy et al., 2011).

Ginger has unique nutritional growing needs. According to Nagarajan and Pillai (1979), ginger needs a steady supply of N, K, PH, Mg, and lesser so, Ca (cited in Parthasarathy et al., 2011). Aerial plant portions begin to decrease nutrient uptake around 80 days into growth. The rhizomes consistently pull nutrients right up until harvest (Parthasarathy et al., 2011; Singh et al., 2012). Ginger is targeted by specialized insects and diseases including root knot nematode, rhizome rot and bacterial wilt (Parthasarathy et al., 2011).

The ginger cultivation described above mainly touches upon international ginger production and that which occurs in Hawaii. In the continental United States, with a much cooler, less tropical, and shorter growing season than many of the tropical countries which have been growing ginger for ages (Parthasarathy et al., 2011; Singh et al., 2012), ginger cultivation has taken on a relatively new and reportedly successful niche market—that of the growing, processing, and sale of "baby" or "young" or "fresh" ginger. Fresh ginger has been rising in popularity in the United States.

In 1999, farm owners Melissa Bahret and Chrissy Steinberg of Old Friends Farm in Amherst, Massachusetts, began to grow USDA certified organic ginger (with rhizomes from Biker Dude Organic Ginger Farm in Pahoa, Hawaii) in unheated hoop-houses (Bahret, 2007). The farmers applied for Sustainable Agriculture Research and Education (SARE) grants to study and compare different cultivation methods and during the process, discovered a high demand from customers for the finished product, young ginger. Young or fresh ginger is a byproduct of the northeast's climate and location—as the growing season is too short in the northeast to harvest mature ginger. However, when ginger fingers are planted in the spring in northern continental U.S. and allowed to grow for about 152 days—the harvested product is a creamy white, juicy and supple rhizome which is vastly different from its mature, dried counterpart (Bahret, 2007). Fresh ginger sells for a higher price than its dried, mature version—at up to $25 per pound. Chefs, breweries, herbalists, and other food and beverage producers are buying this product, along with market customers and CSA farm members.

8.13 Culinary Uses

Ginger has been used to both spice foods and as a health tonic for thousands of years. Dried ginger, which is the form of ginger primarily used for food flavoring, is known for its spicy, pungent aroma and flavor (Attokaran, 2017). Ginger is used to flavor baked goods, candies, teas and juices, and savory dishes (Attokaran, 2017; Lim, 2016). Candied ginger is a popular remedy for many travelers experiencing motion sickness, dizziness, or nausea. Most of the ground and dried ginger sold worldwide is for the purpose of culinary food preparation (Nair, 2013). In Ayurvedic medicine, a drink of fresh ginger, dried ginger, rock salt, black pepper, and long pepper is administered to alleviate sinus pressure, treat fevers, and to clear phlegm (Nair, 2019). In traditional Chinese medicine, a tea of fresh ginger is used to aid circulatory health. Ginger is a cultural superfood and powerhouse offering medicinal benefits along with its globally popular flavor and spice (Zanteson, 2020). Below are two recipes featuring ginger and other nutritional standouts.

Ginger and Turmeric Smoothie (Adapted from Baker, 2020) Ingredients:

- 1 ripe banana
- ¼ tsp. cayenne powder
- 1/2 Tbsp fresh ginger (peeled // 1 small knob yields ~1/2 Tbsp)
- 1/4 tsp. ground turmeric
- ¼ tsp. cinnamon
- ¼ cup fresh cilantro
- 1/2 cup carrot juice
- 1 Tbsp lemon juice
- 1 cup unsweetened almond or oat milk

Directions:

1. Add smoothie ingredients to a blender or food processor and blend on high until you reach desired consistency (creamy is best).

Homemade Pickled Ginger (Splawn, 2020) Ingredients:

- 8 ounces (1/2 pound) fresh baby ginger
- 1 cup unseasoned rice vinegar
- 1/4 cup sugar (or more to taste)
- 1 teaspoon kosher salt

Directions:

1. Wash and scrub ginger well to remove any remaining bits of dirt or soil. Use a spoon to scrape off any thick or papery bits of skin. If using mature ginger, you will want to fully peel it.
2. Thinly slice ginger across the grain using a vegetable peeler or mandoline (please watch your fingers)! You want the ginger to be as paper thin as possible, and I found the peeler to be the most effective way to do this.
3. Place sliced ginger in a bowl. Pour 2 cups of boiling water over ginger and let sit for 5 minutes. If using mature ginger, you might want to blanch the ginger in a pot of boiling water for 5 to 10 minutes to soften it further.
4. Drain well, then pack ginger into one pint jar or two half-pint (8 oz) mason jars. Be sure jars are thoroughly washed or, even better, sanitized in boiling water prior to using.
5. In a saucepan, bring vinegar, sugar, and salt to a simmer, stirring until sugar is completely dissolved.
6. Pour hot liquid over ginger in jars. Secure lids and allow the jars to cool to room temperature, then refrigerate. The pickled ginger, which is ready to eat after several hours, will keep in the refrigerator for up to six months.

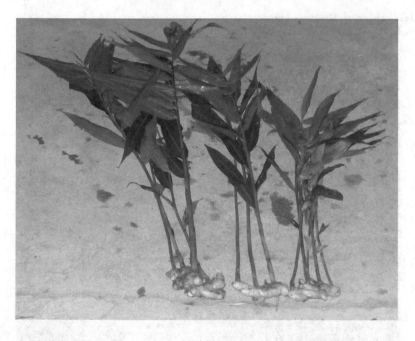

Ginger with stalks
Sengai Podhuvan, CC BY-SA 3.0 <https://creativecommons.org/licenses/by-sa/3.0>, via Wikimedia Commons

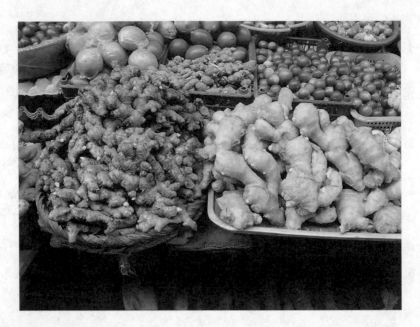

Ginger in Market, Hainan, China
Anna Frodesiak, Public domain, via Wikimedia Commons

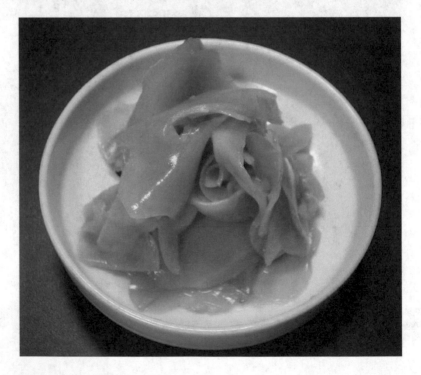

Gari, pickled ginger, Japan
DoWhile, Public domain, via Wikimedia Commons

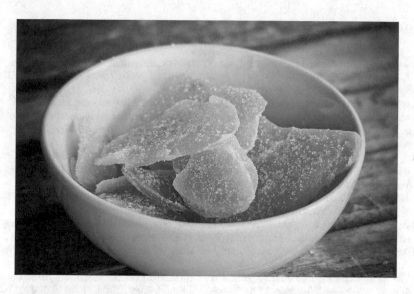

Candied Ginger
Sweetlouise on Pixabay

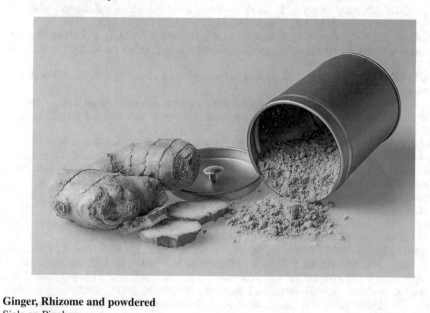

Ginger, Rhizome and powdered
Siala on Pixabay

References

Akbar, S. (2020). Zingiber officinale Rosc. (Zingiberaceae): Syns.: Amomum zingiber L.; A. angustifolium Salisb. In *Handbook of 200 medicinal plants* (pp. 1957–1997). [Online]. Springer International Publishing.

Attokaran, M. (2017). *Natural food flavors and colorants*. John Wiley & Sons, Incorporated.

Azam, A. (2014). Ginger components as new leads for the design and development of novel multi-targeted anti-Alzheimer's drugs: A computational investigation. *Drug Design, Development and Therapy*. [Online], 82045–82059.

Babu, K. N., & Ravindran, P. N. (2004). *Ginger: The Genus Zingiber*. Taylor & Francis Group, Baton Rouge. Available from: ProQuest Ebook Central. [22 December 2020]. Created from csu on 2020-12-22 05:52:07.

Bahret, M. (2007). *Greenhouse Cultivation in the Northeast Part II*, viewed 28 October, 2020. https://northeast.sare.org/news/ginger-an-ancient-crop-in-the-new-world/

Baker, M. (2020). *Carrot ginger turmeric smoothie*. blog post, viewed November 27, 2020. https://minimalistbaker.com/carrot-ginger-turmeric-smoothie/#wprm-recipe-container-35567

Buhner, S. (2013). *Herbal antivirals: Natural remedies for emerging and resistant viral infections*. Storey.

Butt, M. S., & Sultan, M. T. (2011). Ginger and its health claims: Molecular aspects. *Critical Reviews in Food Science and Nutrition, 51*(5), 383–393. https://doi.org/10.1080/10408391003624848

Grzanna, R., Lindmark, L., & Frondoza, C. G. (2005). Ginger – An herbal medicinal product with broad anti-inflammatory actions. *Journal of Medicinal Food*. [Online], *8*(2), 125–132.

Lim, T. (2016). Zingiber officinale. In *Edible medicinal and non-medicinal plants* (pp. 469–560). Springer International Publishing. https://doi.org/10.1007/978-3-319-26065-5_21

Mao, Q.-Q., Xu, X.-Y., Cao, S.-Y., Gan, R.-Y., Corke, H., Beta, T., & Li, H.-B. (2019). Bioactive compounds and bioactivities of ginger (Zingiber officinale Roscoe). *Foods, 8*(6), 185. https://doi.org/10.3390/foods8060185

Nair, K. (2013). *The agronomy and economy of turmeric and ginger: The invaluable medicinal spice crops*. Elsevier.

Nair, K. (2019). *Turmeric (Curcuma longa L.) and ginger (Zingiber Officinale Rosc.) – World's invaluable medicinal spices: The agronomy and economy of turmeric and ginger*. Springer International Publishing AG.

Odle, C. (2014). Ginger. In *The Gale Encyclopedia of Alternative Medicine* (Vol. 2, pp. 995–997).

Parthasarathy, V. A., Srinivasan, V., Nair, R. R., Zachariah, T. J., Kumar, A., Prasath, D., & Janick, J. (2011). Ginger: botany and horticulture. In *Horticultural Reviews*. [Online] (pp. 273–388). John Wiley & Sons, Inc.

Rupasinghe, V., & Gunathilake, K. D. P. P. (2015). Recent perspectives on the medicinal potential of ginger. *Botanics*. [Online], *5*(default), 55–63.

Sang, S. (2020). Precision research on ginger: The type of ginger matters. *Journal of Agricultural and Food Chemistry, 68*(32), 8517–8523. [Online].

Sharifi-Rad, M., Varoni, E., Salehi, B., Sharifi-Rad, J., Matthews, K., Ayatollahi, S., Kobarfard, F., Ibrahim, S., Mnayer, D., Zakaria, Z., Sharifi-Rad, M., Yousaf, Z., Iriti, M., Basile, A., & Rigano, D. (2017). Plants of the genus Zingiber as a source of bioactive phytochemicals: From tradition to pharmacy. *Molecules (Basel, Switzerland)*. [Online], *22*(12), 2145.

Singh, H. P., Parthasarathy, V. A., Kandiannan, K., & Krishnamurthy, K. S. (2012). *Zingiberaceae crops: Present & future cardamom, ginger*. Turmericm and others.

Splawn, M. (2020). "How to pickle ginger" blog post, viewed November 27, 2020. https://www.thekitchn.com/how-to-pickle-ginger-234166

Zanteson, L. (2020). Ginger it Up. *Environmental Nutrition, 43*(4), 8.

Chapter 9
Oily Fish

Michael Pagliassotti

9.1 Introduction

The fish oil industry can be traced back to the 1770s when cod liver oils were marketed in the United Kingdom as a remedy for rheumatism (H.B. Rice, 2016) (Fig. 9.1). The popularity of fish oil in the twentieth and twenty-first century is largely due to its ability to reduce cardiovascular disease risk factors (Dewailly et al., 2001; Leaf, 2008). The first evidence that fish oil might provide some degree of protection against cardiovascular disease came from the observation that Greenland Eskimos, who consume a diet enriched in fish oil, have a lower mortality from coronary heart disease than do Danes and Americans (Bang et al., 1976; Dyerberg et al., 1978; Leaf, 2008). Fish oil, principally long-chain omega-3 fatty acids (eicosapentaenoic acid (EPA) and docosahexaenoic acid (EPA)), is now sought after for health benefits associated with the brain, eyes, pregnancy, and multiple inflammatory conditions (Angelico & Amodeo, 1978; Augood et al., 2008; Teisen et al., 2020; Thien et al., 1996; H.B. Rice, 2016). In this chapter we will examine the cultural history, health claims, and environmental and marketing issues associated with fish oil. Recipes using oily fish will conclude the chapter.

9.2 Cultural History

Oil-rich fish (or oily fish) are those that have oil distributed through their body, as opposed to white fish, where the main concentration of oils is located in the liver. Although oily fish contain higher levels of oil, they are an essential part of a healthy

M. Pagliassotti (✉)
Colorado State University, Fort Collins, CO, USA
e-mail: michael.pagliassotti@colostate.edu

© The Author(s), under exclusive license to Springer Nature Switzerland AG 2022
J. P. Miller, C. Van Buiten (eds.), *Superfoods*, Food and Health,
https://doi.org/10.1007/978-3-030-93240-4_9

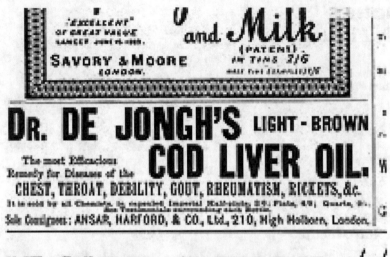

Fig. 9.1 This file is licensed under the Creative Commons Attribution 4.0 International license
L0016974 Text advertisment for Dr. De Jongh's cod liver oil
Credit: Wellcome Library, London. Wellcome Images images@wellcome.ac.uk http://wellco-
meimages.org Text advertisment for Dr. De Jongh's cod liver oil Illustrated London News
Published: 13 April 1895
Copyrighted work available under Creative Commons Attribution only licence CC BY 4.0
http://creativecommons.org/licenses/by/4.0/

diet due to the presence of long-chain omega-3 fatty acids (LC3FAs). Oil-rich fish,
also termed pelagic fish due to the fact that they swim in the pelagic zone or mid- to
surface-waters, include anchovies, eel, herring, mackerel, salmon, swordfish,
and trout.

Anchovies are found in coastal waters of the eastern Atlantic from Norway to
South Africa, as well as in the Mediterranean, Black and Azov seas (Hall, 2005).
Anchovies typically swim in compact schools, feed on plankton during the day, and
then disperse into shallow waters at night. During the Middle Ages, Mediterranean-
based communities with ready access to salt produced anchovies, the most famous
of which was Collioure (Hall, 2005). The only anchovy likely to be found in restau-
rants and stores is the hardy Engraulis encrasicolus, or European anchovy. Although
a small fish, it is characterized by a large jaw and deeply cleft mouth, and thus is
linked to the Spanish name, boqueron or big mouth.

No fish is more generally and widely known than the common eel and none has
been involved in more mystery (Fig. 9.2). According to John Wyatt Greenlee, a
Medieval historian and overseer of an eel-history twitter account, eels have been

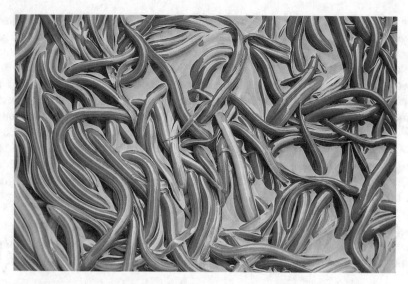

Fig. 9.2 This file is licensed under the Creative Commons Attribution-Share Alike 3.0 Unported, 2.5 Generic, 2.0 Generic and 1.0 Generic license

Description	**English: Eel in Vietnam**
	Nederlands: Alen in Vietnam
Date	**11 October 2013**
Source	**Own work**
Author	**Peter van der Sluijs**

used to pay rent to the Normans in the eleventh century, make wallets, clothes and wedding bands, and as a remedy to stop bloody noses (where eel skin was snorted) (Waxman, 2020). The most commonly consumed eels, anguillas, spend infancy as a leaf-shaped larva called a leptocephalus in the ocean, spend adulthood in fresh water and then return to the ocean to spawn and die. Interestingly, spawning occurs in the Sargasso Sea and thus some eels travel thousands of miles from their fresh water habitat to the Sargasso Sea (Casey, 2010).

Herring is an oily silver-colored fish found in the North Atlantic, Baltic and North Sea. In the twelfth to fourteenth centuries herring was abundant in the Baltic waters around southern Sweden. In the fifteenth century herring spawning grounds moved towards the Netherlands and later into the North Sea. The Herring trade eventually moved towards the west coast of Norway and the northern part of the UK in the nineteenth century (Walsh, 1986). Young Herring caught by the Dutch between mid-May and the end of June are called Hollandse Nieuwe and are prepared using traditional techniques including cleaning, gutting and salting while leaving the pancreas in place to assist with ripening. Surstromming, which means "sour Herring" is a staple food in some regions of Sweden. Pickled Herring has been a staple food in Northern Europe since Medieval times. A kipper, traditionally served for breakfast in the United Kingdom, is a whole Herring with guts and gills removed, split down the back from head to tail, cured in a light brine and cold smoked at an air temperature not higher than 30 °C typically over smoldering oak.

Mackerel (Fig. 9.3) encompass over 30 different species and belong to the Scrombridae family (which also includes tuna and bonito). Common coastal species include the Atlantic Spanish mackerel (east coast of North America), Atlantic mackerel (north Atlantic), chub mackerel (Pacific ocean), and Chilean jack mackerel (south Pacific). Mackerel is an important fish both culturally and economically along the southern coast of Norway, where it represents the taste of summer for Norwegians. Mackerel can live up to 25 years, are characterized by a striking green and blue color, with a number of tiger-like irregular cross bands along its back (Darlina et al., 2011).

Atlantic salmon has been fished throughout most of the European coast since Paleolithic times. Nonetheless, Atlantic salmon are now absent from ~80% of the rivers in North America that they were once found in. Pacific salmon are of the

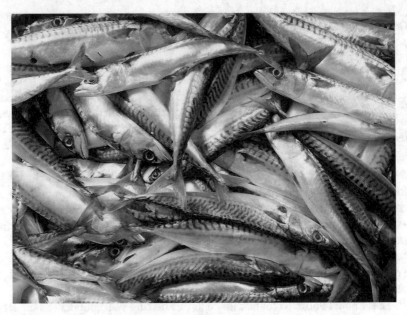

Fig. 9.3 This file is licensed under the Creative Commons Attribution-Share Alike 3.0 Unported license

English: Mackerel at a market in The Hague, Netherlands. Nederlands: Makreel op de Haagse Markt, Den Haag, Nederland.	
Date	**3 April 2015**
Source	**Own work**
Author	**Vincent van Zeijst**

family Oncorhynchus and fishing of this species in North America began ~9000 years ago (Lichatowich, 2001). The importance of salmon is highlighted by the presence of regulations to protect salmon stocks since the year 1030 and its appearance in indigenous art as a food. The most pressing threats to salmon include loss of genetic variation and habitat deterioration. Currently, there are more hatchery raised than wild stock salmon in the Pacific Northwest (Lichatowich, 2001; Longo et al., 2014).

Swordfish (Xiphias gladius or broadbills) are found widely in tropical and temperate parts of the Atlantic, Pacific, and Indian Oceans. They are ectothermic but have organs next to their eyes to heat their eyes and brain. Trout are closely related to salmon and char species and primarily live in freshwater lakes and rivers. However, some trout, for example steelhead trout, can spend 2–3 years at sea before returning to fresh water to spawn. In Australia, the rainbow trout was introduced in 1894 from New Zealand (Nicoletti, 2017).

9.3 Fish Oil: Current State of Research and Health Claims

Jorn Dyerberg and Hans Olaf Bang provided the first evidence that oily fish may have preventative effects on coronary artery disease when they compared the diets of Greenland Eskimos, who are characterized by a low mortality rate when compared to Americans and Danes, with that of Americans and Danes (Bang et al., 1976; Dyerberg et al., 1978; Leaf, 2008). The fat content of the Eskimo diet was largely derived from whale blubber, seal fat, and some oily fish fat, fat sources that contain high amounts of the long chain, omega-3 fatty acids (LC3FAs) eicosapentaenoic acid (EPA) and docosahexaenoic acid (DHA). Table 9.1 provides information on LC3FA content in oily fish. In this section, we will focus on research that has investigated health claims associated with LC3FAs that involve asthma, cardiovascular disease, cognitive performance & mental health, pregnancy outcomes, and psoriasis.

Table 9.1 LCFA content of fish

Fish	Long-chain omega-3 fatty acid content
Eel	838 mg/100 g
Swordfish	1101 mg/100 g
Trout	1370 mg/100 g
Atlantic mackerel	1422 mg/100 g
Sardines	1692 mg/100 g
Bluefin tuna	1710 mg/100 g
Anchovies	2113 mg/100 g
Herring	2217 mg/100 g
Salmon	2585 mg/100 g

9.3.1 LC3FA Supplements

LC3FA supplementation is the most widely used approach to examine the health benefits of fish oil, particularly when examining benefits associated with cardiovascular disease. In 2012, ~8% of adults in the US reported consuming a fish oil dietary supplement within the past 30 days (Clarke et al., 2015; Siscovick et al., 2017). Nonprescription and prescription preparations of LC3FAs exist and can contain fish oil, EPA with and without DHA, varying chemical forms and additional essential nutrients such as vitamins D and E (Siscovick et al., 2017).

9.3.2 Asthma

Asthma is an inflammatory condition that results in narrowing of the bronchial tubes and has increased worldwide over the past three decades in both children and adults (Asher et al., 2006; Yang et al., 2013). Although laboratory-based studies suggest that LC3FAs may reduce risk of asthma, systematic reviews of the epidemiologic evidence have resulted in inconclusive results (Calder, 2006; Hardy et al., 2016; Yang et al., 2013). The analysis of 4 studies where associations between fish or LC3FA intake and risk of asthma were examined (996 cases from 12,481 children and 1311 cases from 82,533 adults) found a beneficial effect of both fish intake and fish oil consumption on risk for childhood asthma but no beneficial effect in adults (Yang et al., 2013). Why is there a discrepancy between laboratory-based and epidemiologic studies? In many cases this discrepancy likely involves the dose of fish or fish oil. For example, Bisgaard and colleagues found that EPA and DHA supplementation in the third trimester of pregnancy reduced the risk of asthma during the first 5 years of a child's life (Bisgaard et al., 2016; Ramsden, 2016). The dose of EPA and DHA provided (2.4 g/d) in this trial was ~10 times higher than the average US intake.

9.3.3 Cardiovascular Disease

Cardiovascular disease is characterized by multiple physiologic events such as chronic progression of stable plaque, plaque instability, acute plaque rupture, thrombosis, and ischemia. This complexity presents a considerable challenge when trying to assess the efficacy of a food or food supplement to provide a health benefit. Current scientific opinion supports the notion that a reduction in mortality (~10% reduction) due to cardiovascular disease is a likely benefit of LC3FA therapy (Leaf, 2008; Mori, 2014; Ridker, 2016; Siscovick et al., 2017). In addition, LC3FAs have been shown to benefit several cardiovascular disease risk factors including lipid levels, blood pressure, and inflammation (Appel et al., 1993; Geleijnse et al., 2002; Lee et al., 1985; Mori, 2014; Mori et al., 1999). For the general population incorporation of at least two oily fish meals per week as part of a healthy diet that includes increased consumption of fruits and vegetables, and reduced salt intake has been recommended (Mori, 2014). Recommendations for patients with cardiovascular disease include 1 gram daily LC3FA supplements and in hypertriglyceridemic patients up to 4 grams per day (Mori, 2014).

9.3.4 Cognitive Performance and Mental Health

Definitive conclusions regarding the ability of LC3FAs to positively influence cognitive performance or mental health cannot be made (Danthiir et al., 2014; Del Brutto et al., 2016; Hansen et al., 2015; van de Rest et al., 2009). Recent studies support these equivocal findings. A randomized trial in which children (n = 232) were randomly assigned to receive lunch meals consisting of either herring/mackerel or chicken/lamb/beef three times per week for 16 weeks did not find differences in changes in mental health or sleep between the two groups (Hysing et al., 2018). Similar findings were observed in which 4–6 year old children received either Atlantic salmon or meat three times per week for 16 weeks (Demmelmair et al., 2019). In contrast, cognitive performance was improved in children (8–9 years old, n = 199) who were randomly assigned to receive 300 g/d of oily fish compared to those who received poultry (Teisen et al., 2020). In older adults, some evidence exists that suggest high doses of oily fish intake (8–9 servings per week over a prolonged period) may provide some degree of protection against cognitive decline (Del Brutto et al., 2016).

9.3.5 Pregnancy Outcomes

DHA is the primary long chain omega-3 fatty acid in brain tissue, representing 10–20% of the total fatty acid composition (Mcnamara & Carlson, 2006). The amount of DHA rises sharply during gestation therefore it is logical to speculate that fish oil supplementation during pregnancy may provide beneficial effects to offspring. There is no definitive evidence that oily fish intake or fish oil supplementation during pregnancy direct impacts cognitive function in offspring (Gale et al., 2008; Judge et al., 2007; Markhus et al., 2020; Tofail et al., 2006). Likewise, studies that have examined the effects of fish intake or fish oil supplementation during pregnancy on anthropometric outcomes have produced equivocal results (Bisgaard et al., 2013). Nonetheless, fish oil supplementation from the 24th week of pregnancy (2.4 g/d) has led to a higher body mass index in offspring from 0 to 6 years of age but not an increased risk of obesity at age 6 (Vinding et al., 2018). In addition, fish oil supplementation (2.4 g/d) during the third trimester of pregnancy was associated with prolonged gestation and increased size for gestational age in a recent randomized control trial (Vinding et al., 2019).

9.3.6   Psoriasis

Two recent systematic analyses of randomized control trials (RCTs) suggest that fish oil supplementation alone does not significantly influence psoriasis. In one, 3 RCTs encompassing 337 participants were examined. In this analysis, fish oil supplementation did not significantly reduce the severity of psoriasis (Yang & Chi, 2019). In the second, 18 RCTs involving 927 participants were examined. In this analysis, fish oil supplementation alone did not significantly impact psoriasis area or severity. However, when fish oil was combined with conventional treatments a positive effect on severity and lesion area was observed (Chen et al., 2020).

9.4   Issues: Contaminants and Sustainability & Fish Oil Markets

9.4.1   Contaminants

Seafood can be a source of contaminants including mercury, methylmercury and selenium (Fig. 9.4). As a general rule lower trophic level oily fish (lower down the food chain), such as salmon, herring, anchovies and sardines, have high concentrations of EPA and DHA and relatively low concentrations of mercury and other contaminants. In contrast, higher trophic oily fish, such as swordfish, will typically have higher concentrations of mercury and other contaminants when compared to lower trophic oily fish (Gribble et al., 2016). A randomized control trial during pregnancy (n = 137 pregnant women) examined whether consumption of Atlantic cod (a fish with relatively low levels of methylmercury) influenced total hair mercury. One group received 400 g of cod fillets per wk. whereas the control group remained on their habitual diet for 16 wks (gestational weeks 20–36). Cod consumption led to non-significant increases in mercury and did not lead to an increase in the number of subjects exceeding the US EPA reference dose (Naess et al., 2020). In another study, chemical contaminants were assessed, including arsenic, cadmium, mercury and lead in five commonly consumed marine fish species (including sardines and mackerel) in Angola. None of the species exceeded the European Union maximum levels for cadmium, mercury and lead and potential consumer exposure to cadmium and methylmercury was low (Moxness Reksten et al., 2020). Some studies have found that heavy metals can be higher in the bones of fish compared to flesh and that canning, depending on the metal type and reduction of moisture loss, can enhance metal levels by 35–80% (Galitsopoulou et al., 2012). A major scientific gap in our understanding of contaminants in fish and human exposure to these contaminants is that fish tissue concentrations of both contaminants and nutrients across a range of species and geographic regions have been rarely assessed.

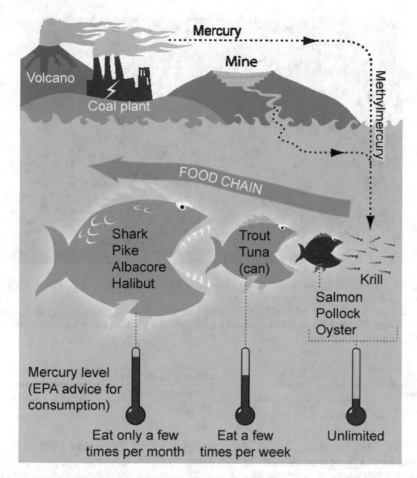

Fig. 9.4 This file is licensed under the Creative Commons Attribution 3.0 Unported license

This figure shows some common sources of mercury, the conversion to toxic methylmercury and the outline of EPA consumption recommendations for certain types of fish based on mercury levels.

Source	Original text: From www.groundtruthtrekking.org: • Source URL: http://www.groundtruthtrekking.org/Graphics/Large/MercuryFood Chain-01.png • Source page: http://www.groundtruthtrekking.org/Graphics/MercuryFoodChain.html
Author	Bretwood Higman, ground truth trekking.

9.4.2 Sustainability and Fish Oil Markets

Pauly and colleagues perhaps said it best, "Fisheries have rarely been sustainable. Rather, fishing has induced serial depletions, long masked by improved technology, geographic expansion and exploitation of previously spurned species lower in the

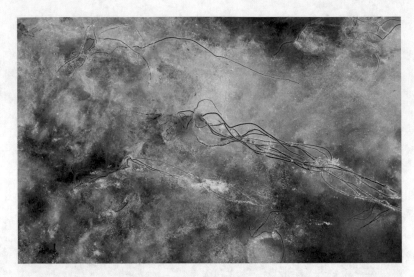

Fig. 9.5 This file is made available under the Creative Commons CC0 1.0 Universal Public Domain Dedication
Marine algae in Gullmarsfjorden at Sämstad, Lysekil Municipality, Sweden. The long hairy strands of Dead Man's Rope (*Chorda filum*) are about 1 m (3.3 ft) high and the bottom is covered with soft blanket weed (*Cladophora glomerata*)

Date	12 July 2019, 10:17:28
Source	Own work
Author	W.carter

food web" (Pauly et al., 2002). The current market for EPA- and DHA-oils has grown by double-digits over the last 30 years. In 2012, it was estimated that consumers spent more than $26 billion dollars on products containing EPA and DHA oils worldwide (H.B. Rice, Rice & Ismail, 2016). The harvest of low trophic species such as anchovy, sardines, and mackerel, represents the main source of LC3FAs used in aqua and animal feeds, health supplements, pharmaceuticals and other products including functional foods (Kitessa et al., 2014).Solutions to this tug of war between consumer interest and fish depletion are currently being examined. For example, single cell organisms such as algae (Fig. 9.5) and genetically modified yeast that can produce LC3FAs are now in commercial production (Kitessa et al., 2014; Lam & Lee, 2012). In addition, genetic engineering to allow oilseed crops to produce LC3FAs has received considerable attention (Nichols et al., 2010). Issues of supply and demand for fish oil require consideration of sustainability as well as alternative sources of LC3FAs. Certainly, ethical and safety considerations will be an important component of the assessment of the feasibility of these alternative sources.

9.5 Recipes

Fresh is best when it comes to choosing oil-rich fish because the fish oil contained within them can deteriorate rapidly. Look for fish that are still stiff, with bright, clear eyes with little to no smell. Oily fish must be stored in as cool a place as possible and eaten quickly, ideally on the day of purchase. Arrange it in a single layer on a tray and keep cool by covering the fish with ice. Oil-rich species freeze well for a short period of time: gut or fillet them, pack into freezer bags as whole fish (or two portions at a time), extract the air and secure the bag. Defrost the fish for a few hours in the fridge before use.

Oily fish are versatile. They suit grilling, barbecuing, roasting and baking and, in some cases, pan-frying. The natural oils give these fish an intense flavor that pairs well with other strong flavors. Oily fish can also be successfully preserved - smoking, brining and salting are all popular preserving methods.

9.5.1 Anchovy Nicoise Salad

Ingredients (for ~4 servings):

- Dressing – 2 garlic cloves, peeled, finely chopped; 6 fl oz. extra virgin olive oil; 2 tbsp red wine vinegar; pinch sea salt; freshly ground black pepper.
- Salad – 4 free-range eggs; 8 small artichoke hearts, cooked (from a jar is fine); 4 very ripe tomatoes, skinned and quartered; 16 black olives; ½ cucumber, peeled and sliced; 4 spring onions, sliced; handful of fine green beans, topped, tailed and blanched; 1 tin anchovies in olive oil; 1 tbsp freshly chopped chervil; small handful of fresh basil.

Recipe:

1. For the dressing, whisk the garlic and oil together in a bowl.
2. Place the eggs into a saucepan and cover with cold water. Bring up to a boil, switch off heat and leave for 5 minutes. Cool under cold water for 2–3 minutes and the peel the eggs.
3. For the salad, arrange all of the salad ingredients (except the chervil and basil) in a shallow dish. Pour over the vinegar and garlic oil and season to taste with salt and freshly ground black pepper.
4. Finish with a sprinkling of chervil and basil and serve at the table.

Recipe taken from https://www.bbc.co.uk/food/recipes/salade_nicoise_**77851**

9.5.2 Salmon Stir Fry

Ingredients (for ~2 servings): 2 tsp. sesame seeds; 2 skinless salmon fillets; 1 tbsp sunflower or vegetable oil; ½ red onion, cut into 8–10 wedges; 1 red pepper, deseeded and thinly sliced; 1 carrot, thinly sliced; 4 ½ oz. broccoli, cut into small florets; 1 oz. unsalted cashew nuts, halved; 2 garlic cloves, thinly sliced; ½ oz. fresh root ginger, peeled and cut into tiny matchsticks; 1 tsp. cornflour; 1 tsp. dark soy sauce; ½ lemon, grated zest and juice only; ¼ pint vegetable stock.

Recipe:

1. Sprinkle 1 tsp. of sesame seeds over the top of each salmon fillet and press down lightly to help them stick.
2. 2. Heat 1 tsp. of the oil in a large frying pan over medium heat and cook salmon fillets, seed-side down, for 2 minutes, or until lightly brown. Turn and cook the other side for 2 minutes. Flip gently and cook for 1 minute on each side. Transfer to a plate.
3. 3. Return the pan to the heat, add the remaining oil and stir-fry the onion, pepper, carrot and broccoli for 4 minutes. Add the cashews and stir-fry for 2 minutes, or until vegetables are tender-crisp and the nuts are beginning to brown. Add the garlic and ginger and cook for a minute, stirring regularly.
4. 4. Mix the cornflour with the soy sauce and lemon juice in a small bowl. Add the stock to the pan, pour in the lemon mixture and bring to a simmer. Cook for 10–20 seconds, stirring, until the sauce is slightly thickened.
5. 5. Return the salmon to the pan, nestling it among the vegetables, and heat through without stirring for 1–2 minutes. Sprinkle with grated lemon zest and serve.

Recipe taken from: https://www.bbc.co.uk/food/recipes/salmon_stir-fry_63266

References

Angelico, F., & Amodeo, P. (1978). Eicosapentaenoic acid and prevention of atherosclerosis. *Lancet, 2*, 531.

Appel, L. J., Miller, E. R. 3rd, Seidler, A. J., & Whelton, P. K. (1993). Does supplementation of diet with 'fish oil' reduce blood pressure? A meta-analysis of controlled clinical trials. *Archives of Internal Medicine, 153*, 1429–1438.

Asher, M. I., Montefort, S., Bjorksten, B., Lai, C. K., Strachan, D. P., Weiland, S. K., Williams, H., & group, I. P. T. S. (2006). Worldwide time trends in the prevalence of symptoms of asthma, allergic rhinoconjunctivitis, and eczema in childhood: ISAAC phases one and three repeat multicountry cross-sectional surveys. *Lancet, 368*, 733–743.

Augood, C., Chakravarthy, U., Young, I., Vioque, J., De Jong, P. T., Bentham, G., Rahu, M., Seland, J., Soubrane, G., Tomazzoli, L., Topouzis, F., Vingerling, J. R., & Fletcher, A. E. (2008). Oily fish consumption, dietary docosahexaenoic acid and eicosapentaenoic acid intakes, and associations with neovascular age-related macular degeneration. *The American Journal of Clinical Nutrition, 88*, 398–406.

Bang, H. O., Dyerberg, J., & Hjoorne, N. (1976). The composition of food consumed by Greenland Eskimos. *Acta Medica Scandinavica, 200*, 69–73.

Bisgaard, H., Vissing, N. H., Carson, C. G., Bischoff, A. L., Folsgaard, N. V., Kreiner-Moller, E., Chawes, B. L., Stokholm, J., Pedersen, L., Bjarnadottir, E., Thysen, A. H., Nilsson, E., Mortensen, L. J., Olsen, S. F., Schjorring, S., Krogfelt, K. A., Lauritzen, L., Brix, S., & Bonnelykke, K. (2013). Deep phenotyping of the unselected COPSAC2010 birth cohort study. *Clinical and Experimental Allergy, 43*, 1384–1394.

Bisgaard, H., Stokholm, J., Chawes, B. L., Vissing, N. H., Bjarnadottir, E., Schoos, A. M., Wolsk, H. M., Pedersen, T. M., Vinding, R. K., Thorsteinsdottir, S., Folsgaard, N. V., Fink, N. R., Thorsen, J., Pedersen, A. G., Waage, J., Rasmussen, M. A., Stark, K. D., Olsen, S. F., & Bonnelykke, K. (2016). Fish oil-derived fatty acids in pregnancy and wheeze and asthma in offspring. *The New England Journal of Medicine, 375*, 2530–2539.

Calder, P. C. (2006). n-3 polyunsaturated fatty acids, inflammation, and inflammatory diseases. *The American Journal of Clinical Nutrition, 83*, 1505S–1519S.

Casey, C. (2010). Spaghetti with eyes: The story of the eel, from a continuing series on revolting creatures. *Slate Magazine*.

Chen, X., Hong, S., Sun, X., Xu, W., Li, H., Ma, T., Zheng, Q., Zhao, H., Zhou, Y., Qiang, Y., Li, B., & Li, X. (2020). Efficacy of fish oil and its components in the management of psoriasis: a systematic review of 18 randomized controlled trials. *Nutrition Reviews, 78*, 827–840.

Clarke, T. C., Black, L. I., Stussman, B. J., Barnes, P. M., & Nahin, R. L. (2015). Trends in the use of complementary health approaches among adults: United States, 2002–2012. *National Health Statistics Reports*, 1–16.

Danthiir, V., Hosking, D., Burns, N. R., Wilson, C., Nettelbeck, T., Calvaresi, E., Clifton, P., & Wittert, G. A. (2014). Cognitive performance in older adults is inversely associated with fish consumption but not erythrocyte membrane n-3 fatty acids. *The Journal of Nutrition, 144*, 311–320.

Darlina, M. N., Masazurah, A. R., Jayasankar, P., Jamsari, A. F., & Siti, A. M. (2011). Morphometric and molecular analysis of mackerel (Rastrelliger spp) from the west coast of Peninsular Malaysia. *Genetics and Molecular Research, 10*, 2078–2092.

Del Brutto, O. H., Mera, R. M., Gillman, J., Zambrano, M., & Ha, J. E. (2016). Oily fish intake and cognitive performance in community-dwelling older adults: the Atahualpa project. *Journal of Community Health, 41*, 82–86.

Demmelmair, H., Oyen, J., Pickert, T., Rauh-Pfeiffer, A., Stormark, K. M., Graff, I. E., Lie, O., Kjellevold, M., & Koletzko, B. (2019). The effect of Atlantic salmon consumption on the cognitive performance of preschool children – A randomized controlled trial. *Clinical Nutrition, 38*, 2558–2568.

Dewailly, E., Blanchet, C., Lemieux, S., Sauve, L., Gingras, S., Ayotte, P., & Holub, B. J. (2001). n-3 fatty acids and cardiovascular disease risk factors among the Inuit of Nunavik. *The American Journal of Clinical Nutrition, 74*, 464–473.

Dyerberg, J., Bang, H. O., Stoffersen, E., Moncada, S., & Vane, J. R. (1978). Eicosapentaenoic acid and prevention of thrombosis and atherosclerosis? *Lancet, 2*, 117–119.

Gale, C. R., Robinson, S. M., Godfrey, K. M., Law, C. M., Schlotz, W., & O'callaghan, F. J. (2008). Oily fish intake during pregnancy – Association with lower hyperactivity but not with higher full-scale IQ in offspring. *Journal of Child Psychology and Psychiatry, 49*, 1061–1068.

Galitsopoulou, A., Georgantelis, D., & Kontominas, M. (2012). The influence of industrial-scale canning on cadmium and lead levels in sardines and anchovies from commercial fishing centres of the Mediterranean Sea. *Food Additives & Contaminants. Part B, Surveillance, 5*, 75–81.

Geleijnse, J. M., Giltay, E. J., Grobbee, D. E., Donders, A. R., & Kok, F. J. (2002). Blood pressure response to fish oil supplementation: Metaregression analysis of randomized trials. *Journal of Hypertension, 20*, 1493–1499.

Gribble, M. O., Karimi, R., Feingold, B. J., Nyland, J. F., O'hara, T. M., Gladyshev, M. I., & Chen, C. Y. (2016). Mercury, selenium and fish oils in marine food webs and implications for human health. *Journal of the Marine Biological Association of the United Kingdom, 96*, 43–59.

Hall, C. (2005). Homage to the anchovy coast. *Smithsonian Magazine*.

Hansen, A. L., Dahl, L., Olson, G., Thornton, D., Grung, B., & Thayer, J. F. (2015). A long-term fatty fish intervention improved executive function in inpatients with antisocial traits and a history of alcohol and drug abuse. *Scandinavian Journal of Psychology, 56*, 467–474.

Hardy, M. S., Kekic, A., Graybill, N. L., & Lancaster, Z. R. (2016). A systematic review of the association between fish oil supplementation and the development of asthma exacerbations. *SAGE Open Medicine, 4*, 2050312116666216.

Hysing, M., Kvestad, I., Kjellevold, M., Kolden Midtbo, L., Graff, I. E., Lie, O., Hurum, H., Stormark, K. M., & Oyen, J. (2018). Fatty fish intake and the effect on mental health and sleep in preschool children in FINS-KIDS, a randomized controlled trial. *Nutrients, 10*.

Judge, M. P., Harel, O., & Lammi-Keefe, C. J. (2007). Maternal consumption of a docosahexaenoic acid-containing functional food during pregnancy: benefit for infant performance on problem-solving but not on recognition memory tasks at age 9 mo. *The American Journal of Clinical Nutrition, 85*, 1572–1577.

Kitessa, S. M., Abeywardena, M., Wijesundera, C., & Nichols, P. D. (2014). DHA-containing oilseed: A timely solution for the sustainability issues surrounding fish oil sources of the health-benefitting long-chain omega-3 oils. *Nutrients, 6*, 2035–2058.

Lam, M. K., & Lee, K. T. (2012). Microalgae biofuels: A critical review of issues, problems and the way forward. *Biotechnology Advances, 30*, 673–690.

Leaf, A. (2008). Historical overview of n-3 fatty acids and coronary heart disease. *The American Journal of Clinical Nutrition, 87*, 1978S–1980S.

Lee, T. H., Hoover, R. L., Williams, J. D., Sperling, R. I., Ravalese, J. 3rd, Spur, B. W., Robinson, D. R., Corey, E. J., Lewis, R. A., & Austen, K. F. (1985). Effect of dietary enrichment with eicosapentaenoic and docosahexaenoic acids on in vitro neutrophil and monocyte leukotriene generation and neutrophil function. *The New England Journal of Medicine, 312*, 1217–1224.

Lichatowich, J. (2001). *Salmon without Rivers: A history of the Pacific Salmon crisis*. Island Press.

Longo, S. B., Clausen, R., & Clark, B. (2014). Capitalism and the commodification of Salmon. *Monthly Review*.

Markhus, M. W., Hysing, M., Midtbo, L. K., Nerhus, I., Naess, S., Aakre, I., Kvestad, I., Dahl, L., & Kjellevold, M. (2020). Effects of two weekly servings of cod for 16 weeks in pregnancy on maternal iodine status and infant neurodevelopment: Mommy's food, a randomized controlled trial. *Thyroid*.

McNamara, R. K., & Carlson, S. E. (2006). Role of omega-3 fatty acids in brain development and function: Potential implications for the pathogenesis and prevention of psychopathology. *Prostaglandins, Leukotrienes, and Essential Fatty Acids, 75*, 329–349.

Mori, T. A. (2014). Omega-3 fatty acids and cardiovascular disease: epidemiology and effects on cardiometabolic risk factors. *Food & Function, 5*, 2004–2019.

Mori, T. A., Bao, D. Q., Burke, V., Puddey, I. B., & Beilin, L. J. (1999). Docosahexaenoic acid but not eicosapentaenoic acid lowers ambulatory blood pressure and heart rate in humans. *Hypertension, 34*, 253–260.

Moxness Reksten, A., Joao Correia Victor, A. M., Baptista Nascimento Neves, E., Myhre Christiansen, S., Ahern, M., Uzomah, A., Lundebye, A. K., Kolding, J., & Kjellevold, M. (2020). Nutrient and chemical contaminant levels in five marine fish species from Angola – The EAF-Nansen Programme. *Food, 9*.

Naess, S., Kjellevold, M., Dahl, L., Nerhus, I., Midtbo, L. K., Bank, M. S., Rasinger, J. D., & Markhus, M. W. (2020). Effects of seafood consumption on mercury exposure in Norwegian pregnant women: A randomized controlled trial. *Environment International, 141*, 105759.

Nichols, P. D., Petrie, J., & Singh, S. (2010). Long-chain omega-3 oils-an update on sustainable sources. *Nutrients, 2*, 572–585.

Nicoletti, J. (2017). On this day; trout arrive in Australia. *Australian Geographer*.

Pauly, D., Christensen, V., Guenette, S., Pitcher, T. J., Sumaila, U. R., Walters, C. J., Watson, R., & Zeller, D. (2002). Towards sustainability in world fisheries. *Nature, 418*, 689–695.

Ramsden, C. E. (2016). Breathing easier with fish oil – A new approach to preventing asthma? *The New England Journal of Medicine, 375*, 2596–2598.

Rice, H. B., & Ismail, A. (2016). Fish oils in human nutrition: History and current status. In *Fish and fish oil in health and disease prevention*. Academic Press.

Ridker, P. M. (2016). Fish consumption, fish oils, and cardiovascular events: Still waiting for definitive evidence. *The American Journal of Clinical Nutrition, 104*, 951–952.

Siscovick, D. S., Barringer, T. A., Fretts, A. M., Wu, J. H., Lichtenstein, A. H., Costello, R. B., Kris-Etherton, P. M., Jacobson, T. A., Engler, M. B., Alger, H. M., Appel, L. J., Mozaffarian, D., & American Heart Association Nutrition Committee of the Council on Lifestyle and Cardiometabolic Health; Council on Epidemiology and Prevention; Council on Cardiovascular Disease in the Young; Council on Cardiovascular and Stroke Nursing; and Council on Clinical Cardiology. (2017). Omega-3 polyunsaturated fatty acid (fish oil) supplementation and the prevention of clinical cardiovascular disease: A science advisory from the American Heart Association. *Circulation, 135*, e867–e884.

Teisen, M. N., Vuholm, S., Niclasen, J., Aristizabal-Henao, J. J., Stark, K. D., Geertsen, S. S., Damsgaard, C. T., & Lauritzen, L. (2020). Effects of oily fish intake on cognitive and socio-emotional function in healthy 8-9-year-old children: the FiSK junior randomized trial. *The American Journal of Clinical Nutrition, 112*, 74–83.

Thien, F. C., Woods, R. K., & Walters, E. H. (1996). Oily fish and asthma – A fishy story? Further studies are required before claims can be made of a beneficial effect of oily fish consumption on asthma. *The Medical Journal of Australia, 164*, 135–136.

Tofail, F., Kabir, I., Hamadani, J. D., Chowdhury, F., Yesmin, S., Mehreen, F., & Huda, S. N. (2006). Supplementation of fish-oil and soy-oil during pregnancy and psychomotor development of infants. *Journal of Health, Population, and Nutrition, 24*, 48–56.

van de Rest, O., Spiro, A., 3rd, Krall-Kaye, E., Geleijnse, J. M., de Groot, L. C., & Tucker, K. L. (2009). Intakes of (n-3) fatty acids and fatty fish are not associated with cognitive performance and 6-year cognitive change in men participating in the veterans affairs normative aging study. *The Journal of Nutrition, 139*, 2329–2336.

Vinding, R. K., Stokholm, J., Sevelsted, A., Sejersen, T., Chawes, B. L., Bonnelykke, K., Thorsen, J., Howe, L. D., Krakauer, M., & Bisgaard, H. (2018). Effect of fish oil supplementation in pregnancy on bone, lean, and fat mass at six years: Randomised clinical trial. *BMJ, 362*, k3312.

Vinding, R. K., Stokholm, J., Sevelsted, A., Chawes, B. L., Bonnelykke, K., Barman, M., Jacobsson, B., & Bisgaard, H. (2019). Fish oil supplementation in pregnancy increases gestational age, size for gestational age, and birth weight in infants: a randomized controlled trial. *The Journal of Nutrition, 149*, 628–634.

Walsh, G. P. (1986). The history of the herring and with its decline the significance to health. *Medical Hypotheses, 20*, 133–137.

Waxman, O. B. (2020). Keeping it Eel: How one historian is using twitter and medieval factoids to help endangered animals. *Time Magazine*.

Yang, S. J., & Chi, C. C. (2019). Effects of fish oil supplement on psoriasis: A meta-analysis of randomized controlled trials. *BMC Complementary and Alternative Medicine, 19*, 354.

Yang, H., Xun, P., & He, K. (2013). Fish and fish oil intake in relation to risk of asthma: A systematic review and meta-analysis. *PLoS One, 8*, e80048.

Chapter 10
Superfood Seeds

Shelby Cox, Kalyn Garcia, and Charlotte Carlson

10.1   Cultural History

Seeds as culinary ingredients have become increasingly popular in recent years primarily due to their nutrient density and potential health benefits. Although their classification as a superfood is a relatively new phenomena, the culinary and medicinal use of seeds dates back to ancient civilizations. Specifically, this chapter will examine three popular seeds: chia, flax, and hemp.

The first documented use of chia seeds dates back to ancient Mesoamerican civilizations. They were primarily used for dietary and medicinal purposes, but some historical evidence suggests chia seeds may have had some importance in artistic and religious practices. They were consumed whole, mixed into drinks, ground into flour, and pressed for oil. Known for their ability to increase stamina and sustain energy, chia seeds remained a staple in the Aztec diet for centuries (Baldivia et al., 2018, pp. 1626–1632).

Flaxseed has been cultivated for thousands of years as a source of oil and fiber for fabric production. In the Middle Ages, flaxseed was believed to have numerous health benefits and—in combination with other ingredients—was used as an antitumor and wound-healing agent; cough, pain and anti-inflammatory remedy; and a treatment for freckles and nail disorders (Goyal et al., 2014, pp. 1633–1653). Because of its perceived health implications, laws and regulations were passed requiring people to consume it regularly (Goyal et al., 2014, pp. 1633–1653). Additionally, Ayurveda, an ancient pseudoscientific medicine system, has used flaxseed in its healing practices for thousands of years and continues to use it today (Goyal et al., 2014, pp. 1633–1653).

S. Cox (✉) · K. Garcia · C. Carlson
Colorado State University, Fort Collins, CO, USA
e-mail: Shelby.cox@colostate.edu

© The Author(s), under exclusive license to Springer Nature Switzerland AG 2022
J. P. Miller, C. Van Buiten (eds.), *Superfoods*, Food and Health,
https://doi.org/10.1007/978-3-030-93240-4_10

Historic findings indicate that the hemp plant, grown in ancient China, is one of mankind's oldest cultivated crops. The hemp plant was mainly used as a food source and in the production of textiles, paper, and medicine (Li, 1974, pp. 437–448). It was believed that consuming the seeds would improve health, strength, and overall life expectancy. Hemp seed was established as one of the five major grains alongside broomcorn, millet, wheat, and soybean. Hemp seed oil was a later development that was used for frying food. It remained an important part of the Chinese diet and culture until other high-yielding grains like wheat, maize and rice were cultivated. As a result, consumption gradually decreased until it eventually became a forgotten food crop (Li, 1974, pp. 437–448).

10.2   Nutritional Research/Health Claims

Chia, flax, and hemp seeds have varying nutrition profiles that impact the health benefits of each. See Table 10.1 for a comparison of nutrients.

10.3   Chia Seeds

The nutrient-rich chia seed is composed of fat (30–33%) carbohydrates (26–41%), dietary fiber (18–30%), protein (15–25%), vitamins, minerals, and antioxidants (Knez Hrnčič et al., 2020, pp. 11). Research shows a possible association between the nutrients in chia seeds and decreased inflammation, protection from free radicals and cancer, and decreased risk of type 2 diabetes and aging disorders.

It is important to note the advantageous fatty acid profile of chia seeds, characterized by high concentrations of both omega-3 and omega-6 fatty acids and a beneficial ratio of omega-3 to omega-6 polyunsaturated fatty acids (PUFA). Dietary intake and/or supplementation of omega-3 fatty acids has been shown to improve cardiovascular function, specifically having an impact on inflammation, peripheral arterial disease (PAD), and coronary events, and improve cognitive functioning in Alzheimer's Disease (Swanson et al., 2012, pp. 1–7). Specific research on chia

Table 10.1 Comparison of nutrient composition for chia, flax, and hemp (per 100 grams)

	Chia	Flax	Hemp
Energy (kcal)	486	534	553
Carbohydrates (g)	42.1	28.9	8.7
Dietary Fiber (g)	34.4	27.3	4
Protein (g)	16.5	18.3	31.6
Fat (g)	30.7	42.2	48.8
Omega-3 (g)	17.8	19.0^2	8.7

U.S. Department of Agriculture; Rodriguez et al. (2010, pp. 489–496)

seeds, inflammation, and cardiovascular disease has found that regular consumption can decrease C-reactive protein, an inflammatory marker, and systolic blood pressure (Vuksan et al., 2007, pp. 2804–2810; Vuksan et al., 2017a, b, pp. 138–146). Furthermore, the antioxidant compounds present in chia seeds, such as tocopherols, phytosterols, carotenoids, and polyphenolic compounds, have been shown to reduce oxidative stress and protect the body from free radicals and cancer (de Falco et al., 2017, pp. 745–760). Additional research shows potential for protection against type 2 diabetes by decreasing hemoglobin A1C and improving glycemic control (Vuksan et al., 2007, pp. 2804–2810, Vuksan et al., 2017a, b, pp. 234–238).

Human clinical trials investigating the effects of chia seed consumption have found mixed results. Overweight women who consumed chia seeds did not have significant improvements in lipoproteins, cholesterol, serum glucose, blood glucose, inflammation, or body mass and composition (Nieman et al., 2012, pp. 700–708). Similar results were found in a group of overweight adults (Nieman et al., 2009, pp. 414–418). However, chia seed intake may improve postprandial glycemia and prolong satiety, with greater benefits at higher amounts (Vuksan et al., 2010, pp. 436–438).

Adequate intake of dietary fiber is important for overall health and reducing the risk for several chronic diseases. However, only 5% of the population meets the recommendations for fiber intake (Quagliani & Felt-Gunderson, 2016, pp. 80–85). Because chia seeds provide a significant amount of fiber (34 grams per 100 gram serving), they have been used in the prophylaxis of several health conditions such as gastrointestinal disorders, heart disease, hypertension, obesity, type 2 diabetes, and certain cancers (Baldivia et al., 2018, pp. 1626–1632).

10.4   Flaxseed

The main components of flaxseed that have health-promoting properties include omega-3 fatty acids, lignans, and fiber. It is the richest plant source for alpha-linoleic acid (ALA) and lignan secoisolariciresinol diglucoside (SDG), both of which offer health benefits. Cardiovascular effects and cancer prevention and treatment are the most researched areas of flaxseed supplementation. Dietary flaxseed has also been associated with positive effects on obesity, type 2 diabetes, inflammation, and oxidative stress (Parikh et al., 2019, pp. 1171).

Dietary flaxseed has a strong ability to regulate cardiovascular disease through its anti-atherogenic effects and anti-inflammatory properties, as well as its potential to improve vascular contractile function (Rodriguez-Leyva et al., 2013, pp. 1081–1089). Regular consumption of whole flaxseed has shown to significantly decrease total cholesterol and low-density lipoprotein (LDL) cholesterol. There is no significant impact on high-density lipoprotein (HDL) cholesterol (Prasad & Dhar, 2016, pp. 141–144; Pan et al., 2009, pp. 288–297). The positive effects on blood lipid profile has been attributed to the anti-inflammatory and antiproliferative properties of ALA. In addition to these attributes, ALA in flaxseed has anti-hypertensive effects, and has been shown to successfully decrease both systolic and diastolic blood pressure (Rodriguez-Leyva et al., 2013, pp. 1081–1089).

Rich compositions of both SDG and ALA are thought to play a role in flaxseed's fight against cancer (Rodriguez-Leyva et al., 2013, pp. 1081–1089). Cancer processes are complex, but lignans have multiple targets and modes of action within the cancer phenotype. Current overall evidence indicates that flaxseed and its lignans provide prophylactic impacts that are effective in the risk reduction and treatment of breast cancer (Mohammadi-Sartang et al., 2018, pp. 125–139). However, flaxseed lignans may have different effects on cancer prevention and treatment depending on the type and stage of cancer (Cunnane et al., 1993, pp. 443–453).

Research suggests that whole flaxseed may also improve diabetes, obesity, insulin resistance, and glycemic control (Cunnane et al., 1993, pp. 443–453; Mandașescu et al., 2005, pp. 502–506). Fiber has the ability to improve inflammatory markers through interfering with several inflammatory pathways. Flaxseed is more likely to reduce systemic inflammatory markers in those with high concentrations of inflammatory factors, such as people with obesity (De Silva & Alcorn, 2019, pp. 68). Dietary fibers, lignans, and omega-3 fatty acids present in flaxseed may have a protective effect against diabetes. Several studies indicate that flaxseed supplementation successfully reduces blood glucose in subjects with type 2 diabetes and prediabetes (Rodriguez-Leyva et al., 2013, pp. 1081–1089). However, further research needs to be conducted to determine if flaxseed is an appropriate dietary intervention to reduce the incidence or delay the development of type 2 diabetes.

Flaxseed supplementation may also be beneficial for certain neural conditions, female hormonal status, gastrointestinal health, and skin health (Rodriguez-Leyva et al., 2013, pp. 1081–1089). Additional research needs to be done to make definitive conclusions and inform dietary recommendations.

10.5   Hempseed

Hempseed has excellent nutritional value. It is rich in essential fatty acids, protein, carbohydrates, vitamins, and minerals. There is limited understanding of the dietary implications of hempseed on human health, but it is an emerging topic. However, there are many animal studies that have shown positive effects of hempseed supplementation.

Hempseed has a desirable omega-6 to omega-3 PUFA ratio that can be beneficial for cardiovascular health, similar to that of flaxseed (Kaushal et al., 2020, pp. 330–338). Recent animal studies show a decreased risk of platelet aggregation and myocardial infarction, plus a better defense against hyperlipidemia by decreasing cholesterol, LDL, and triglyceride levels, as well as lower plaque, fat deposition, and arterial wall damage (Kaushal et al., 2020, pp. 330–338). However, additional research needs to be conducted to indicate the effects hempseed has on cholesterol levels, blood pressure, atherosclerosis, and coronary heart disease in humans (Rodriguez-Leyva & Pierce, 2010, pp. 32).

Hempseed oil may also be a suitable dietary intervention for certain dermatological conditions such as atopic dermatitis and other skin ailments. The beneficial effects are due to the balance and abundance of PUFAs. There are several studies that indicate that hempseed oil can decrease the symptoms and severity of these conditions, but additional research is needed (Reynolds et al., 2019, pp. 1371–1376).

Although the known health benefits are limited, the nutritional makeup and studies in animals suggest hempseed will be a valuable functional food once further human research is conducted.

10.6   Botany/Biology/Chemistry

Salvia hispanica L., more commonly known as chia, is grown primarily for its seeds. They can vary in color ranging from black, grey, or white, to black spotted. The only notable variation is that white seeds are larger, thicker, and broader in comparison to black seeds. The seed color does not significantly affect the nutritional value (Knez Hrnčič et al., 2020, pp. 11). The chia seed, as well as chia leaves, are also used for their oil. This oil, rich in fatty acids, is most often used in the creation of omega-3 supplement capsules in addition to uses as a fragrance or condiment (Coorey et al., 2012, pp. 85–95; Muñoz et al., 2013 pp. 394–408). Chia has a unique mucilage property that can achieve water control and modulate texture across a variety of foods. It can also produce edible films and act as a thickener, foaming, and emulsifying agent (Muñoz et al., 2012 pp. 216–224; Redgwell & Fischer, 2005, pp. 521–535; Muñoz et al., 2012, pp. 511–518). Applications of chia seed use are vast beyond the food industry including use in pest control, animal feed, medical use, and the cosmetics industry due to its nutrient and nutraceutical properties (Muñoz et al., 2013 pp. 394–408). Animal feed applications are of particular interest as various meats and animal products, such as eggs and milk, have improved nutrition profiles when the animals are supplemented with chia seed. For example, chickens fed chia have egg profiles with higher omega-3's and the chicken itself has an improved fatty acid profile, similar to what is seen in pigs, ruminants and fish also fed a chia-enhanced diet (Jamshidi et al., 2019, pp. 1–18). Besides the improvements in nutritional profile on the end product, chia is desirable compared to other seeds due to its minimal effect on the overall flavor of the final products, which is important for their acceptability with consumers. (Jamshidi et al., 2019, pp. 1–18).

Flax is a blue flowering annual herb that produces small flat seeds varying from golden yellow to reddish brown in color (Kajla et al., 2015, pp. 1857–1871). *Linum usitatissimum,* the Latin name of flaxseed translates to "very useful," and rightfully so. Every part of the flax plant is utilized commercially, either directly or after processing (Kajla et al., 2015, pp. 1857–1871). Flaxseed may also be referred to as linseed. These terms are used interchangeably, the main difference being a matter of purpose. Flaxseed is used to describe flax when consumed as food by humans while linseed is used to describe flax when it is used for industrial applications, such as to make linen textiles and paper (Kajla et al., 2015, pp. 1857–1871; Goyal et al., 2014, pp. 1633–1653).

Hemp is grown as an agricultural crop in over 30 nations. Botanically, hemp and marijuana belong to the same species of plant, *Cannabis sativa* L., but genetically, they are quite different. They are both forms of cannabis that can be distinguished by their use, chemical composition, cultivation process, and statutory definition (Johnson, 2019). THC is the dominant psychotropic compound in cannabis. Hemp has a THC threshold of less than 0.3%. Marijuana has no THC threshold. Both hemp and marijuana contain over 60 cannabinoids; however, because hemp contains little to no THC, it is non-psychoactive (Johnson, 2019). Hemp is cultivated for food, dietary supplements, and both therapeutic and industrial purposes, while marijuana is cultivated for recreational and medicinal use.

10.6.1   Social Issues

After spending most of the last three centuries in obscurity, the chia crop rapidly increased in popularity around 2010 (Baldivia et al., 2018, pp. 1626–1632). Chia seeds are now cultivated in Mexico, Guatemala, Australia, Bolivia, Colombia, Peru, Argentina, America, and Europe (Knez Hrnčič et al., 2020, pp. 11). Because heightened demand for chia is a new phenomenon, there are issues in production related to availability and sustainability as an oil product in the global food supply (Mohd Ali et al., 2012, pp. 171956). Historically, there is not enough planting and production of chia to meet the global demand (Mohd Ali et al., 2012, pp. 171956).

Growing awareness of the health benefits of flaxseed has significantly increased the global demand for the crop. Canada is the world's largest producer and exporter of flaxseed; however, it is also grown in the United States, China, India, and Ethiopia. The rise in demand is primarily attributed to the increasing consumption of flaxseed in baked goods, animal feed, and pet food. Because there are numerous applications for each part of the flax plant, it leaves behind virtually no waste. Flaxseed production is sustainable, has a low carbon footprint, and requires minimal water and irrigation.

Until recently, growing hemp was restricted in the United States, making it the largest importer for hemp products. The United States Drug Enforcement Administration (DEA) strictly controlled and regulated hemp production. Under U.S. drug laws, all cannabis varieties, including hemp, were classified as Schedule I controlled substances. Congress expanded the definition of industrial hemp in 2018, further distinguishing it from marijuana, which has allowed for greater hemp cultivation practices (Johnson, 2019). The establishment of a hemp industry in the USA and its rapid expansion in production has considerably impacted global commerce. Rising awareness regarding the dietary advantages of hemp seeds and oil, coupled with cosmetic and personal care uses, is expected to drive market growth over the next eight years, securing a long-term sustainable market for the crop ("Industrial Hemp Market Size," 2020). Hemp production also draws interest due to its low environmental footprint, as hemp can grow in many different agro-ecological conditions, grows quickly, produces high yield, and can be used for carbon sequestration (Rupasinghe et al., 2020, pp. 4078).

10.6.2 Use of Seeds – How to Use/Cook

Chia seeds can be consumed whole, ground, and in the form of flour, gel, and oil (Knez Hrnčič et al., 2020, pp. 11). They can be added or mixed into baked goods, pasta, cereal, and other snack foods. Chia seeds can absorb twelve times their weight in water, making them an appropriate substitute for eggs and fat in recipes. Due to their hydrophilic properties, when chia seeds are immersed in water, the release of mucilage forms a highly viscous solution that can be used as a foam stabilizer, adhesive, emulsifier, or binder (Knez Hrnčič et al., 2020, pp. 11). When used as an egg or oil substitute in baked goods, they are typically used in the form of chia gel.

Because of the high content of omega-3 fatty acids, chia oil can be mixed with butter to improve its lipid profile. Chia oil has a neutral flavor and can be used in most recipes without altering the flavor. Because it is heat-sensitive, chia oil should be used at temperatures below 90 degrees Celsius to preserve its nutritional value (Ghafoor et al., 2020, pp. 127531).

Flaxseed possesses a pleasant, nutty flavor that can be consumed whole, ground into flax meal, and as oil. Flaxseed oil is commonly used in salad dressings, sauces, and dips. Due to its hypersensitivity to heat, oxygen, and light, flaxseed oil is rarely used for cooking, frying or food preparation methods involving heat (Kajla et al., 2015, pp. 1857–1871).

The most prevalent use of flaxseed is in baked goods such as muffins, bagels, bread, buns, biscuits, and pasta (Parikh et al., 2019, pp. 1171). Several multi-grain products such as cereals and snack bars incorporate flaxseed to add a nutty flavor, provide texture, and increase nutritional value. It can also be sprinkled on top of foods to add a crunchy texture. Gelling and binding properties make flaxseed meal a desirable gluten-free thickening agent or egg substitute in baked goods (Kajla et al., 2015, pp. 1857–1871).

Hemp seeds can be consumed whole, but shelled hemp seeds, or hemp hearts, are the most common method of consumption. Additionally, hemp seeds can be made into flour, oil, and milk. Hemp seeds are added to foods to improve the nutritional value and change the sensory properties (Leonard et al., 2020, pp. 282–308). Hemp seeds have successfully been incorporated into various breads, cereals, dairy, and meat products. Hemp hearts are typically consumed sprinkled on top of cereals, salads, yogurt, or blended into smoothies.

Hemp seeds can be a safe option for individuals with food allergies. They can be used as a breadcrumb substitute for those with a gluten sensitivity or blended with water to make hemp seed milk that can be used as a dairy alternative. Toasting hemp seeds brings out their nutty flavor, making them an appropriate alternative for those with nuts allergies. Hemp seed oil can be used for cooking; however, it is heat sensitive. To minimize oxidation, it is best utilized for low-heat cooking or mixed into salad dressings, dips, and other dishes (Leonard et al., 2020, pp. 282–308).

10.6.3   Recipes

Chia Pudding
This chia pudding makes a delicious breakfast full of fiber and unsaturated fats that will keep you satisfied all morning.

Ingredients

- 1 cup milk or milk alternative
- ¼ cup chia seeds
- 1–2 tablespoons maple syrup (to desired sweetness)
- 1 teaspoon vanilla extract

Instructions

1. In a dish, mix all ingredients until combined.
2. Cover and refrigerate overnight (at least 6 hours).
3. The pudding should be thick. If the pudding is thinner than desired, add more seeds, stir, and refrigerate for an additional hour.
4. To serve, enjoy as is or layer in your favorite fresh fruit, jam, or fruit compote, or add fresh mint.

Lemon-Flax Vinaigrette
Making your own salad dressing is easy! This lemon-flax vinaigrette is tasty with any type of salad greens, or you can even use it as a marinade.

Ingredients

- ¼ cup lemon juice
- ¼ cup flaxseed oil
- ¼ cup white balsamic vinegar
- 1 tablespoon Dijon mustard
- 1 clove garlic, minced
- 1 teaspoon honey
- Salt and pepper to taste

Instructions

1. Whisk all ingredients together until well combined.
2. Serve over salad greens, roasted vegetables or poultry and fish.
3. Store in a sealed container in the refrigerator. Oil will separate during storage, shake, or whisk well before each use to re-emulsify.

Hemp Seed Energy Bites

Keep a batch of these hemp seed energy bites in the fridge for grab-and-go snacks during the week. They are high in protein with a hint of sweetness.

Ingredients

- ½ cup creamy nut butter (such as peanut butter or almond butter)
- ¼ cup honey
- ½ cup non-fat dry milk
- ¼ cup rolled old fashioned oats
- ¼ cup crispy rice cereal
- 2 tablespoons hemp hearts
- Optional add-ins: chocolate chips, coconut flakes, chia or flax seed, dried fruit

Instructions

1. In a dish, mix all ingredients until combined.
2. Use your hands to shape mixture into 1-inch balls.
3. Store in an airtight container and refrigerate to keep fresh longer.

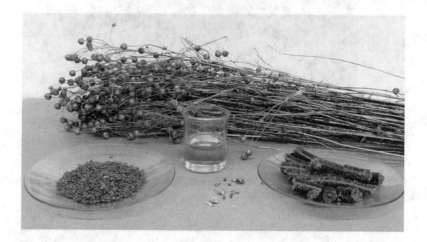

1. From Flax to Linseed Oil- Handwerker, CC BY-SA 3.0 <https://commons.wikimedia.org/wiki/File:From_flax_to_linseed_oil..JPG > via Wikimedia Commons

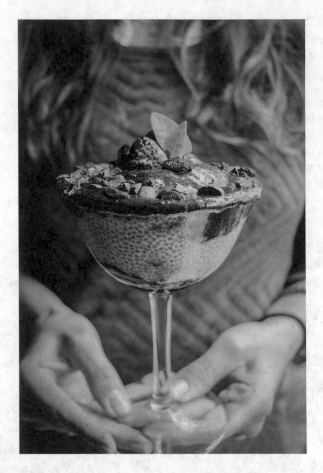

2. Chia Pudding- Sebastián León Prado, CC BY-SA 3.0 <https://unsplash.com/photos/ B2JFNoufa-c > via Wikimedia Commons

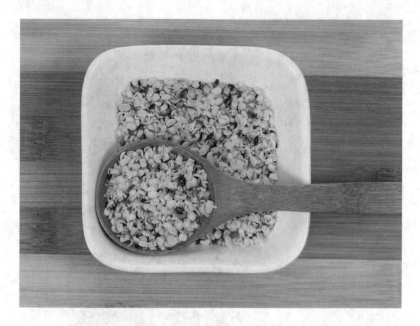

3. Hemp Seeds 1- No attribution required or provided <https://pixabay.com/photos/cannabis-seeds-hemp-raw-bio-3894009/ > via Pixabay

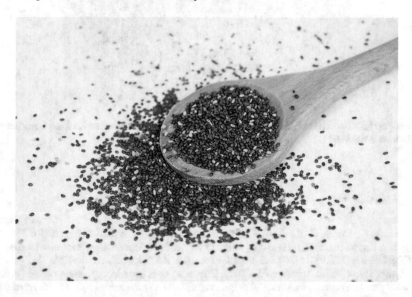

4. Chia Seeds 1- No attribution required or provided < https://pixabay.com/photos/chia-seeds-super-food-eat-healthy-2119771/ > via Pixabay

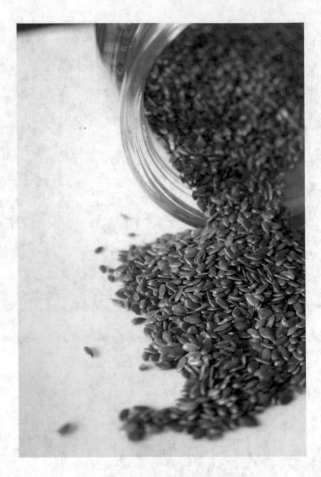

5. Flax Seeds 2- No attribution required or provided. <https://www.pexels.com/photo/brown-seeds-in-a-bottle-691175/> via Pexels

References

Baldivia, A. S., Ibarra, G. R., Torre, R. R. R., López, R. R., & López, A. M. (2018). The chia (Salvia hispanica): Past, present, and future of an ancient Mexican crop. *Australian Journal of Crop Science, 12*(10), 1626–1632. https://doi.org/10.21475/ajcs.18.12.10.p1202

Coorey, R., Grant, A., & Jayasena, V. (2012). Effects of chia flour incorporation on the nutritive quality and consumer acceptance of chips. *Journal of Food Research, 1*(4), 85–95. https://doi.org/10.5539/jfr.v1n4p85

Cunnane, S., Ganguli, S., Menard, C., Liede, A., Hamadeh, M., Chen, Z., ... Jenkins, D. (1993). High α-linolenic acid flaxseed (Linum usitatissimum): Some nutritional properties in humans. *The British Journal of Nutrition, 69*(2), 443–453. https://doi.org/10.1079/BJN19930046

de Falco, B., Amato, M., & Lanzotti, V. (2017). Chia seeds products: an overview. *Phytochemistry Reviews, 16*, 745–760. https://doi.org/10.1007/s11101-017-9511-7

De Silva, S. F., & Alcorn, J. (2019). Flaxseed Lignans as important dietary polyphenols for cancer prevention and treatment: Chemistry, pharmacokinetics, and molecular targets. *Pharmaceuticals (Basel, Switzerland), 12*(2), 68. https://doi.org/10.3390/ph12020068

Ghafoor, K., Ahmed, I. A. M., Özcan, M. M., Al-Juhaimi, F. Y., Babiker, E. E., & Azmi, I. U. (2020). An evaluation of bioactive compounds, fatty acid composition and oil quality of chia (Salvia hispanica L.) seed roasted at different temperatures. *Food Chemistry, 333*, 127531. https://doi.org/10.1016/j.foodchem.2020.127531

Goyal, A., Sharma, V., Upadhyay, N., Gill, S., & Sihag, M. (2014). Flax and flaxseed oil: An ancient medicine & modern functional food. *Journal of Food Science and Technology, 51*(9), 1633–1653. https://doi.org/10.1007/s13197-013-1247-9

Industrial Hemp Market Size, Share & Trends Analysis Report By Product (Seeds, Fiber, Shives), By Application (Animal Care, Textiles, Food & Beverages, Personal Care), And Segment Forecasts, 2020–2027 (2020, February). Grand View Research. https://www.grandviewresearch.com/industry-analysis/industrial-hemp-market

Jamshidi, A. M., Amato, M., Ahmadi, A., Bochicchio, R., & Rossi, R. (2019). Chia (Salvia hispanica L.) as a novel forage and feed source: A review. *Italian Journal of Agronomy, 14*(1), 1–18. https://doi.org/10.4081/ija.2019.1297

Johnson, R. (2019). Defining hemp: A fact sheet. Congressional Research Service, 22 Mar 2019, https://fas.org/sgp/crs/misc/R44742.pdf

Kajla, P., Sharma, A., & Sood, D. R. (2015). Flaxseed—A potential functional food source. *Journal of Food Science and Technology, 52*(4), 1857–1871. https://doi.org/10.1007/s13197-014-1293-y

Kaushal, N., Dhadwal, S., & Kaur, P. (2020). Ameliorative effects of hempseed (Cannabis sativa) against hypercholesterolemia associated cardiovascular changes. *Nutrition, Metabolism, and Cardiovascular Diseases, 30*(2), 330–338. https://doi.org/10.1016/j.numecd.2019.09.006

Knez Hrnčič, M., Ivanovski, M., Cör, D., & Knez, Ž. (2020). Chia seeds (Salvia hispanica L.): An overview-phytochemical profile. *Isolation Methods, and Application Molecules (Basel, Switzerland), 25*(1), 11. https://doi.org/10.3390/molecules25010011

Leonard, W., Zhang, P., Ying, D., & Fang, Z. (2020). Hempseed in food industry: Nutritional value, health benefits, and industrial applications. *Comprehensive Reviews in Food Science and Food Safety, 19*(1), 282–308. https://doi.org/10.1111/1541-4337.12517

Li, H.-L. (1974). An archeological and historical account of cannabis in China. *Economic Botany, 28*(4), 437–448.

Mandaşescu, S., Mocanu, V., Dăscaliţa, A. M., Haliga, R., Nestian, I., Stitt, P. A., & Luca, V. (2005). Flaxseed supplementation in hyperlipidemic patients. *Revista Medico-Chirurgicală a Societăţii de Medici şmi Naturalişmti din Iaşmi, 109*(3), 502–506.

Mohammàdi-Sartang, M., Sohrabi, Z., Barati-Boldaji, R., Raeisi-Dehkordi, H., & Mazloom, Z. (2018). Flaxseed supplementation on glucose control and insulin sensitivity: A systematic review and meta-analysis of 25 randomized, placebo-controlled trials. *Nutrition Reviews, 76*(2), 125–139. https://doi.org/10.1093/nutrit/nux052

Mohd Ali, N., Yeap, S. K., Ho, W. Y., Beh, B. K., Tan, S. W., & Tan, S. G. (2012). The promising future of chia, Salvia hispanica L. *Journal of Biomedicine & Biotechnology, 171956*. https://doi.org/10.1155/2012/171956

Muñoz, L. A., Cobos, A., Diaz, O., & Aguilera, J. M. (2012). Chia seeds: microstructure, mucilage extraction and hydration. *Journal of Food Engineering, 108*(1), 216–224. https://doi.org/10.1016/j.jfoodeng.2011.06.037

Munoz, L. A., Aguilera, J. M., Rodriguez-Turienzo, L., Cobos, A., & Diaz, O. (2012). Characterization and microstructure of films made from mucilage of salvia hispanica and whey protein concentrate. *Journal of Food Engineering, 111*(3), 511–518. https://doi.org/10.1016/j.jfoodeng.2012.02.031

Muñoz, L. A., Cobos, A., Diaz, O., & Aguilera, J. M. (2013). Chia seed (Salvia hispanica): An ancient grain and a new functional food. *Food Reviews International, 29*(4), 394–408. https://doi.org/10.1080/87559129.2013.818014

Nieman, D. C., Cayea, E. J., Austin, M. D., Henson, D. A., McAnulty, S. R., & Jin, F. (2009). Chia seed does not promote weight loss or alter disease risk factors in overweight adults. *Nutrition Research, 29*(6), 414–418.

Nieman, D. C., Gillitt, N., Jin, F., Henson, D. A., Kennerly, K., Shanely, R. A., … Schwartz, S. (2012). Chia seed supplementation and disease risk factors in overweight women: a metabolomics investigation. *Journal of Alternative and Complementary Medicine, 18*(7), 700–708.

Pan, A., Yu, D., Demark-Wahnefried, W., Franco, O. H., & Lin, X. (2009). Meta-analysis of the effects of flaxseed interventions on blood lipids. *The American Journal of Clinical Nutrition, 90*(2), 288–297. https://doi.org/10.3945/ajcn.2009.27469

Parikh, M., Maddaford, T. G., Austria, J. A., Aliani, M., Netticadan, T., & Pierce, G. N. (2019). Dietary flaxseed as a strategy for improving human health. *Nutrients, 11*(5), 1171. https://doi.org/10.3390/nu11051171

Prasad, K., & Dhar, A. (2016). Flaxseed and diabetes. *Current Pharmaceutical Design, 22*(2), 141–144. https://doi.org/10.2174/1381612822666151112151230

Quagliani, D., & Felt-Gunderson, P. (2016). Closing America's Fiber intake gap: Communication strategies from a food and fiber summit. *American Journal of Lifestyle Medicine, 11*(1), 80–85. https://doi.org/10.1177/1559827615588079

Redgwell, R. J., & Fischer, M. (2005). Dietary fiber as a versatile food component: An industrial perspective. *Molecular Nutrition & Food Research, 49*(6), 521–535. https://doi.org/10.1002/mnfr.200500028

Reynolds, K. A., Juhasz, M. L. W., & Mesinkovska, N. A. (2019). The role of oral vitamins and supplements in the management of atopic dermatitis: A systematic review. *International Journal of Dermatology, 58*, 1371–1376. https://doi.org/10.1111/ijd.14404

Rodriguez-Leyva, D., & Pierce, G. N. (2010). The cardiac and haemostatic effects of dietary hempseed. *Nutrition and Metabolism, 7*, 32. https://doi.org/10.1186/1743-7075-7-32

Rodriguez-Leyva, D., Dupasquier, C. M., McCullough, R., & Pierce, G. N. (2010). The cardiovascular effects of flaxseed and its omega-3 fatty acid, alpha-linolenic acid. *The Canadian Journal of Cardiology, 26*(9), 489–496. https://doi.org/10.1016/s0828-282x(10)70455-4

Rodriguez-Leyva, D., Weighell, W., Edel, A. L., LaVallee, R., Dibrov, E., Pinneker, R., Maddaford, T. G., Ramjiawan, B., Aliani, M., Guzman, R., & Pierce, G. N. (2013). Potent antihypertensive action of dietary flaxseed in hypertensive patients. *Hypertension (Dallas, Tex: 1979), 62*(6), 1081–1089. https://doi.org/10.1161/HYPERTENSIONAHA.113.02094

Rupasinghe, H. P., Davis, A., Kumar, S. K., Murray, B., & Zheljazkov, V. D. (2020). Industrial hemp (Cannabis sativa subsp. sativa) as an emerging source for value-added functional food ingredients and nutraceuticals. *Molecules, 25*(18), 4078. https://doi.org/10.3390/molecules25184078

Swanson, D., Block, R., & Mousa, S. A. (2012). Omega-3 fatty acids EPA and DHA: Health benefits throughout life. *Advances in Nutrition, 3*(1), 1–7. https://doi.org/10.3945/an.111.000893

U.S. Department of Agriculture, Agricultural Research Service. Food Data Central. (2019). fdc.nal.usda.gov

Vuksan, V., Whitham, D., Sievenpiper, J. L., Jenkins, A. L., Rogovik, A. L., Bazinet, R. P., Vidgen, E., & Hanna, A. (2007). Supplementation of conventional therapy with the novel grain Salba (Salvia hispanica L.) improves major and emerging cardiovascular risk factors in type 2 diabetes: results of a randomized controlled trial. *Diabetes Care, 30*(11), 2804–2810. https://doi.org/10.2337/dc07-1144

Vuksan, V., Jenkins, A. L., Dias, A. G., Lee, A. S., Jovanovski, E., Rogovik, A. L., & Hanna, A. (2010). Reduction in postprandial glucose excursion and prolongation of satiety: possible explanation of the long-term effects of whole grain Salba (Salvia Hispanica L.). *European Journal of Clinical Nutrition, 64*(4), 436–438.

Vuksan, V., Jenkins, A. L., Brissette, C., Choleva, L., Jovanovski, E., Gibbs, A. L., Bazinet, R. P., Au-Yeung, F., Zurbau, A., Ho, H. V. T., & Duvnjak, L. (2017a). Salba-chia (Salvia hispanica L.) in the treatment of overweight and obese patients with type 2 diabetes: A double-blind randomized controlled trial. *Nutrition, Metabolism, and Cardiovascular Diseases, 27*(2), 138–146. https://doi.org/10.1016/j.numecd.2016.11.124

Vuksan, V., Choleva, L., Jovanovski, E., Jenkins, A. L., Au-Yeung, F., Dias, A. G., Ho, H. V. T., Zurbau, A., & Duvnjak, L. (2017b). Comparison of flax (Linum usitatissimum) and Salba-chia (Salvia hispanica L.) seeds on postprandial glycemia and satiety in healthy individuals: a randomized, controlled, crossover study. *European Journal of Clinical Nutrition, 71*, 234–238. https://doi.org/10.1038/ejcn.2016.148

Chapter 11
Tea

Tiffany Weir

11.1   Cultural History

Medicine, political symbol, pinnacle of hospitality, and even a philosophy - from its ancient Chinese roots (Okakura, 1906) to the Boston Tea Party and the Opium Wars, a beverage made from the leaves of *Camellia sinensis L.*, has left a distinctive mark on our world. The origins of tea stretch beyond the reach of history and into the realm of legend. One popular story recounts how leaves from a tea tree accidentally fell into a cup of warm water being served to the emperor, Shen Nong. Being pleased with the aroma, the emperor drank the beverage, marking the introduction of tea to the Chinese nobility. Another legend relates how the "divine farmer", Shennong, accidentally poisoned himself after testing wild plants in search of edible leaves and grains. As he lay dying, a tea leaf drifted down from a tree and into his mouth, reviving him. In reality, tea cannot reverse the effects of poisons, but Lu Yu's eighth century monograph "The Classic of Tea" serves as record of some of its early medicinal uses (Yu & Demi Hitz, 1974).

Popularization of the use of tea as a beverage in China may have stemmed from its cultivation and use by Buddhist monks, who found that the caffeine in tea helped them stay awake through long hours of meditation. By the Tang Dynasty (581–618 CE) tea preparation had become an artform and tea drinking was enjoyed by all social classes in China (Yu & Demi Hitz, 1974). Over 1000 years ago, tea began to spread throughout Asia along a caravan route, referred to as the Tea Horse Road, which brought tea, salt, silk and other goods into the Himalayas in exchange for horses (Freeman & Ahmed, 2011). Through this original route, tea was brought into Tibet and Nepal, and from there it continued to spread to India and Burma. Buddhist monks brought tea to Japan; and their ritualistic method of preparing

T. Weir (✉)
Colorado State University, Fort Collins, CO, USA
e-mail: tiffany.weir@colostate.edu

© The Author(s), under exclusive license to Springer Nature Switzerland AG 2022   141
J. P. Miller, C. Van Buiten (eds.), *Superfoods*, Food and Health,
https://doi.org/10.1007/978-3-030-93240-4_11

powdered green tea (matcha) by whisking it into water is still part of the traditional Japanese tea ceremony. In the 1500s, the Portuguese- and later the Dutch- established sea trade routes with China, bringing tea to western Europe.

It wasn't until the seventeenth century, when King Charles II of England married Catherine of Braganza, a Portuguese princess, that tea drinking became popularized amongst the British aristocracy (Martin, 2007). It was nearly another century, before tea became affordable for the masses and widely consumed by citizens across the British Empire. This demand for tea, and the desire for Britain to control its trade and production is inextricably linked to the Empire's expansion. England's East India Company (EIC), originally established in 1600 by Queen Elizabeth I to monopolize the British spice trade (Robins, 2006), was a major player- first through trade domination and later through political power. About 90% of the EIC's profits came from the tea trade, and the EIC helped Parliament fund the Carnatic Wars, cementing Britain's territorial foothold in India and eventually helping them establish British-controlled tea plantations (Webster, 2011).

In the mid 1820–1840s, prior to establishment of tea plantations in India, China was the only commercial source of tea. The Chinese had no need for products made or grown outside their borders and demanded payment in silver bullion. This trade deficit with China and their demand for silver became a heavy financial burden on British business interests. However, there was a demand in China for illegal opium, which was produced in parts of India that were under British control. The EIC, through the use of proxy companies, began to smuggle opium into China to generate silver, which in turn was used to fund the British tea addiction (Webster, 2011). Chinese authorities, wishing to put a stop to the illegal opium trade, seized and destroyed twenty thousand tons of British-owned opium, which angered members of the British Parliament and sparked the First Opium War (1839–1842). Two British warships defeated a fleet 29 Chinese junks, and the ensuing Treaty of Nanjing ceded Hong Kong to Britain and allowed the opening of new trading ports.

Around the time of the Carnatic Wars in India, the British government was also struggling to maintain political control over the American colonies. The colonists were heavily taxed on British commodities, and although most of these taxes were later repealed, taxation of tea through the Townshend Act persisted (Ketchum, 2002). This resulted in American boycotts of tea imported by the EIC, while illegal smuggling fulfilled the colonies demand for tea. In an effort to regain the market and help financially buoy the struggling EIC, Parliament passed the Tea Act of 1773 (Higginbotham & Labaree, 1965). This allowed the EIC to export their tea duty-free while still taxing colonists through the Townshend Act. Colonists viewed this as an attempt at political subjugation and began turning EIC ships away at several ports. However, several EIC ships-the *Dartmouth, Eleanor*, and *Beaver*- made it into the port of Boston. There they were met by armed militia who prevented them from unloading their cargo, boarded the ships, and dumped forty thousand kilograms of tea into the Boston Harbor (Ketchum, 2002). British repercussions for the Boston Tea Party further enraged colonists and provided the impetus sparking the American Revolution.

Today, tea is the second most popular beverage in the world, and its ties to British colonialism are often forgotten by modern tea drinkers. Instead, tea has taken on its own significance and characteristics in each culture where it has been adopted. Richly spiced black teas are frequently consumed in India, while the British favor bergamot-spiced Earl Grey, often with milk and sugar. Tibetans consume fermented brick teas with yak's milk and salt to create mind-body balance, and Americans often consume their teas cold. However, one commonality amongst tea drinkers around the world is the perception that tea consumption imparts specific health benefits. These purported benefits and their underlying chemistry will be covered in the next few sections.

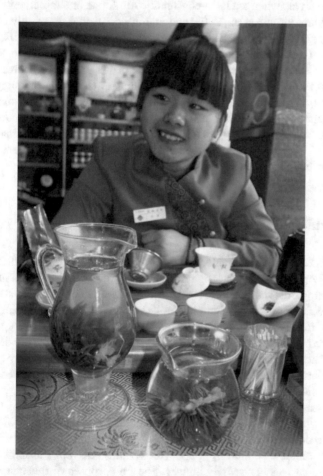

"Flower" tea tasting at a tea shop. Nanjing, China; credit Tiffany Weir

11.2   Nutrition Information

When consumed as an infusion, with no added sugars or milk, tea is basically devoid of the standard essential nutrients. An 8 oz. brew of green tea can have around 0.4 g carbohydrates, 0 g fat, and 0.1 g protein, and 0 g of dietary fiber, according to the USDA's National Nutrient Database. Tea leaves contain several vitamins, such as vitamin C, folate, β-carotene (a precursor to vitamin A), and thiamine; however, very low levels of these vitamins transfer from the tea leaves to the brewed beverage. For example, a recent study examining teas available through U.S. retail venues reported an average of 45 mg/100 g of vitamin C in leaves, but only ~0.5 mg/100 g in the brewed tea (Somanchi et al., 2021). Likewise, there are reports of reduced serum folate levels when tea is co-consumed with foods or supplements containing folic acid (Alemdaroglu et al., 2008) and in individuals that frequently consume tea (Shiraishi et al., 2010), suggesting that tea may reduce the bioavailability of dietary folate. On the other hand, many minerals found in tea leaves are also found in the brewed tea. One study reported that four cups of tea provided as much as 1% of daily calcium and phosphorus requirements and up to 5–6% of magnesium and potassium requirements (Schwalfenberg et al., 2013). Unfortunately, toxic elements that accumulate in tea leaves can also be found in appreciable amounts in some brewed teas. Some of the samples tested for beneficial minerals also had unacceptable levels of toxic aluminum and lead, particularly when leaves were allowed to steep for more than 3 minutes (Schwalfenberg et al., 2013).

11.3   Health Claims

Despite limited nutritional value, health claims surrounding tea consumption are common. These health claims range from benefits for weight loss and management to preventing cardiovascular disease and diabetes. The health benefits of tea have largely been demonstrated in pre-clinical animal models and are mainly attributed to a suite of bioactive phytochemicals, such as catechins and thearubigins. As discussed in the next section, the concentrations of these components are dependent on agronomic factors, as well as how the tea leaves are processed. Many anti-oxidant and anti-inflammatory phytochemicals are generally higher in green teas compared to black teas. As a result, more studies done in human populations have focused on the health benefits of green tea consumption, and there is limited translational evidence as to whether black teas have similar effects. In addition, several pre-clinical studies have demonstrated unique phytochemical components and a wide array of physiologic effects mediated by "dark" (fermented) teas, but translational data for these benefits are also extremely limited. For the purposes of this chapter, we will only examine health effects that have been demonstrated in human observational or intervention studies and that are associated with consumption of brewed teas or whole tea powders (such as matcha) rather than supplements made of extracted tea components.

Weight Loss Green tea, a minimally processed tea rich in catechins and often higher in caffeine, is most often associated with weight loss. Although there is a good deal of heterogeneity, both in methods and results of studies examining green tea effects on weight loss, the number of published studies is sufficient to warrant several systematic reviews and meta-analyses. One meta-analysis of five random controlled trials examining consumption of varying amounts (range: 300 mg tea water extracts-4 cups of brewed tea/day) of green or fermented (Pu-ehr) teas in individuals with metabolic syndrome reported a modest decrease in BMI (-0.72 kg/ m^2) in their pooled analysis, and no significant overall reduction in weight compared to the control groups (Zhong et al., 2015). However, a more recent meta-analysis, comprised of 25 placebo-controlled clinical trials in obese or overweight individuals, reported that green tea supplementation resulted in significant but modest (average of <2 kg) weight loss, with individuals that were classified as obese (BMI > 30 kg/m^2) showing greater reduction in weight (~2.5 kg) (Lin et al., 2020). This meta-analysis included trials conducted in several Asian and European countries as well as in the United States and Brazil. This is important to note as a recent literature review observed that the effects of green tea on weight loss were more consistent and pronounced in interventions conducted on Asian subjects compared to Caucasians (Huang et al., 2014). In each of these meta-analyses, greater weight loss and BMI reduction were observed when tea was administered concomitant with a diet management plan. Thus, while green tea consumption does not appear to be a magic bullet for dieters, it may enhance weight loss when consumed in conjunction with other interventions, such as caloric restriction and increased physical activity.

Cardiovascular Disease Cardiovascular disease is a collection of conditions that include coronary heart disease (CHD), stroke, high blood pressure, and heart failure. A recent meta-analysis that included 24 studies with a total of nearly 1700 participants concluded that a short-term intervention with green tea resulted in significantly reduced systolic and diastolic blood pressure. However, the reductions noted were < 2 mm/Hg, which is unlikely to be clinically significant (Xu et al., 2020). Similar conclusions were drawn from a meta-analysis of 14 trials looking at short term intervention (4–24 weeks) with green or black teas, where it was reported that tea consumption had no significant effect on either blood pressure or circulating blood lipids (Igho-Osagie et al., 2020). However, interpretation of these studies are limited by a lack of standardized doses provided to participants. An examination of 22 prospective studies that included >850,000 individuals, one of the largest meta-analyses to date, demonstrated that consumption of at least 3 cups of tea/day was associated with ~25% reduced risk of CHD, heart failure, and a 20% reduced risk of stroke- although it did not reduce mortality among those who had strokes (Zhang et al., 2015). These results warrant a closer examination to determine whether cardiovascular benefits are associated with a specific type of tea (black or green) and to determine the required doses for reducing disease risk.

Diabetes Although there are numerous studies examining the impact of tea consumption on diabetes risk and maintenance, the results are equivocal. Several meta-analyses suggest that benefits, if any, for diabetes prevention are modest. One meta-analysis of nine cohort studies, including over 300,000 individuals, suggested that tea drinkers were not protected from developing diabetes, although there was a modest risk reduction when tea consumption exceeded 4 cups/day (Chen et al., 2020). In a Chinese cohort of .5 M individuals, there was a modest reduction (~8%) in the risk of developing type 2 diabetes in daily tea drinkers, particularly those that drank green tea or had been consuming tea for >30 years (Nie et al., 2021). However, another large Chinese cohort study including more than 100,000 adults, suggested that tea consumption was associated with a significant increase in risk of developing diabetes in both men and women (Liu et al., 2018). Tea consumption also appears to have limited effects on regulating glucose metabolism in diabetic individuals. A meta-analysis of six studies looking at markers of glucose metabolism in diabetic individuals showed that compared to placebo, green tea consumption did not improve glycosylated hemoglobin (HbA1c), fasting glucose or insulin, and homeostatic model assessment for insulin resistance (HOMA-IR) (Yu et al., 2017). However, another meta-analysis suggested that C-reactive protein, a circulating marker of inflammation, was reduced in diabetic green tea consumers compared to individuals that did not drink tea, suggesting that diabetics may experience some benefits from tea consumption (Asbaghi et al., 2019). Like other meta-analyses looking at tea-related health outcomes, it is difficult to identify a precise dose required for specific cardiovascular benefits. Therefore, translation of these results to clinical recommendations for improving health is limited.

Health Benefits of Dark Teas As discussed in the following section, dark teas are produced by microbial fermentation and aging of tea leaves. This process results in altered metabolite profiles in the brewed tea when compared to non-fermented tea leaves (Keller et al., 2013a). The health benefits of consuming dark teas have mainly been explored in animal models, but the few existing human studies on dark teas are promising (Lin et al., 2021). For example, an observational study of individuals with hypercholesterolemia showed that 120 days of Fuzhuan tea consumption (brewed using 5 grams tea leaves) improved lipid parameters (Fu et al., 2011). Similar results were seen in mildly obese, hypercholesterolemic individuals consuming Pu-ehr tea for 4 weeks (Jensen et al., 2016). Mechanistically, these effects may be due to the anti-microbial activity of theabrownin in these teas against bile salt hydrolyzing microbes in the gut. Loss of these microbes influences bile acid metabolism in the gut, ultimately suppressing intestinal farnesoid X receptor (FXR), which signals the liver to increase bile acid synthesis (Huang et al., 2019). There is also some evidence for dark-tea mediated improvements in glucose homeostasis in humans. In a population of healthy adults, 2 grams of Pu-ehr tea dissolved in water attenuated post-prandial glucose levels (Takeda et al., 2019). Furthermore, a retrospective cross-sectional study in >17,000 Chinese individuals also suggested that daily dark tea drinkers had a 46% reduced risk of developing Type 2 diabetes compared to non-tea drinkers, while there was no reduction in risk for daily green or black tea drinkers (Chen et al., 2020). Although the overall body of evidence supporting benefits of dark teas is still quite small, they may prove to be the true superfoods among teas, largely due to their unique microbial and phytochemical profiles.

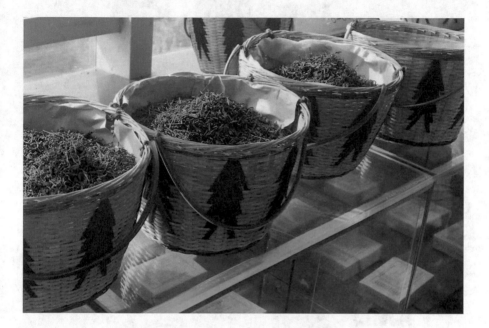

Baskets of loose leaf fermented Fu tea. Hunan Provence, China; credit Tiffany Weir

11.4 Botany/Biology/Chemistry/Biochemistry

Despite the numerous varieties of commercially available tea, the botanical diversity is somewhat limited. Commercial tea leaves are picked from *Camellia sinensis* (L.) plants, grown as a low bush and maintained in a perpetual vegetative state. The plant itself is heterogenous, with continuous variation in vegetative characteristics and a high degree of physiologic plasticity, making it difficult to classify distinct varieties (Banerjee, 1992). As a result, there are local landraces of tea, but only two recognized varieties: *C. sinensis* var. *sinensis* (L.) and *C. sinensis* var. *assamica* (Masters) Kitamura (Banerjee, 1992; Kitamura, 1950). The *sinensis* variety are shorter and slower growing with narrow, erect, serrated dark green leaves, while the *Assam* variety are taller, faster growing, and have broad, horizontal leaves that are non-serrated and lighter green (Kitamura, 1950).

For the casual consumer, botanical differences among tea plants are much less important a feature than the method of processing. Consumers can choose from white/yellow, green, oolong, black/red, and dark teas (Fig. 11.1).

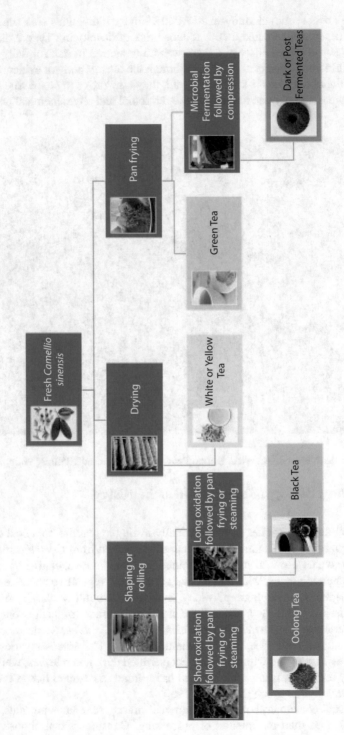

Fig. 11.1 Processing steps and fpr different tea classifications

There are also quality designations, such as "orange pekoe". Orange pekoe is a grade of black tea leaf, reserved for the newest flush of leaves and the apical bud. Within the orange pekoe grade, there are additional distinctions such as "flowery orange pekoe" which means it includes the buds, and "golden flowery orange pekoe" which has a higher ratio of buds to leaves. Tea bags typically contain the remnants left over from processing higher quality leaves, and their flavors are less full and nuanced than whole leaf varieties. Tea colors are assigned based on the appearance of the beverage and correspond to how the leaves are processed. For example, white tea contains only the bud and the immature first leaves, which are pan-fired to inactivate the enzyme, polyphenol oxidase, prior to drying. Green teas are made from slightly older leaves, but are also processed immediately to prevent oxidation, while oolong is partially oxidized and black/red teas are fully oxidized (Weir et al., 2012). Dark teas are a class of microbially-fermented tea, with Pu-erh being the most widely known. The process by which they are made varies from region to region but may include pile fermentation, inoculation with fungal spores, and controlled aging (Weir et al., 2012). Unlike other types of tea, dark teas often gain value with age. Each of these processing methods imparts unique flavors and aromas to the brewed beverage and influences the phytochemical content and health attributes associated with the various tea types.

Camellia sinensis contains several bioactive phytochemicals that are transferred to the beverage during the brewing process. These include caffeine, flavonoids- such as the catechins, theaflavins, and thearubigins, and L-theanine, a non-protein amino acid (Kc et al., 2020). Although numerous environmental and agronomic factors impact concentrations of these compounds in the leaves, post-harvest processing has the greatest impact on the amounts of these compounds present in the consumed beverage (Kim et al., 2011; Lin et al., 2003). White and green teas have the highest amount of the flavan-3-ols, or catechins, in particular epigallocatechin gallate (EGCG). However, polyphenol oxidase, which remains active in oolong and black teas, oxidizes the catechins, facilitating their condensation into dimers (theaflavins) and polymers (thearubigins). Therefore, oolong and black teas have fewer catechins, but higher theaflavins and thearubigins (Lin et al., 2003). There are also several other flavonoids found in tea which are not impacted by processing, such as quercetin and kaempferol. Black teas typically have more caffeine than green and oolong teas, although this is mainly due to differences in water temperature and brewing time rather than caffeine content of the leaves. In contrast, green teas are associated with higher levels of L-theanine. Dark teas are less-well studied, but have chemical profiles similar to black teas with the addition of organic acids and other metabolites produced during fermentation (Keller et al., 2013b; Ping et al., 2020).

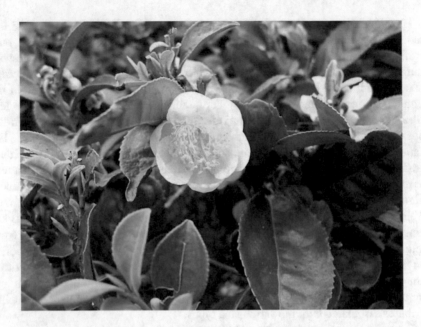

Kristian Frisk Creative Commons Attribution-Share Alike 2.0 Flower in a tea plant at a Darjeeling Tea plantation

11.5 Social and Environmental Issues

Like many agricultural products, particularly those grown on plantations, tea cultivation is not without its social and environmental issues. In terms of the environmental impacts, many tea plantations have displaced rainforests, reducing biodiversity and wildlife habitat. These monoculture plantations reduce land fertility and require high levels of chemical inputs for sustainable production. Tea processing, such as drying leaves, is energy intensive and often requires firewood that is collected from local forests, further increasing deforestation and leaving the land vulnerable to degradation and mudslides in areas where monsoon weather occurs. Efforts to mitigate these issues include a move toward permaculture in tea plantations, organic production, and improved processing infrastructure. Certification such as Rainforest Alliance can help consumers identify teas that make an effort to mitigate environmental impacts.

Poor conditions and low wages paid to workers are pervasive social issues in the industry, and despite rising market prices, profit going to tea producers has remained stagnant for the past 30 years (Turner & Webb, 2014). Large tea companies purchase minimally processed bulk tea for further processing and packaging, and along with retailers, they capturing ~86% of the value added compared to <1% of the total profits that go to tea pickers (Hilary & Dromey, 2010). For example, according to a 2014 report, a tea picker in Assam was paid 89 rupees/day, while the legal daily minimum wage for unskilled workers in Assam was 158.54 rupees (Long, 2014). This equates to below a living wage and leaves children, particularly girls, vulnerable to human traffickers. Initiatives by certification agencies such as Fairtrade International, The Sustainable Trade Initiative, UTZ Certified, Rainforest Alliance, as well as standards set by certain companies, such as Unilever, are working towards improving wage and benefit auditing and supporting livelihoods of workers in ways that are socially and economically relevant. These include maternity leave, written contracts, and agreements for overtime as well providing plantations and co-ops with certification premiums that can be used to support education and healthcare for workers or improve farm conditions and processing infrastructure. Conscientious consumer can influence the flow of money within the industry by purchasing certified teas (ie. Fairtrade), sourcing teas directly from plantations or smallholder cooperatives, and buying single origin, minimally processed teas.

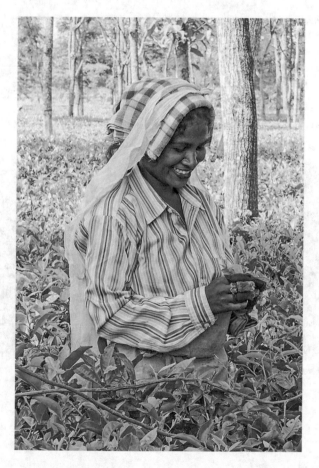

Woman harvesting tea, West Bengal, India Bernard Gagnon
Creative Commons Attribution-Share Alike 4.0 Quality image

11.6 Recipes

Teas can be incorporated into various types of sweet and savory dishes. Green teas are often used for desserts, providing a clean, delicate flavor to mochi, biscuits, or ice creams. Darker teas, like black and oolong, are often the base of "milk teas", including chai and Thai teas. They can also be used as a meat and fish marinade, adding depth and complexity to savory dishes. However, tea is more commonly consumed as a hot beverage and to experience the unique flavors and aromas of different teas, proper brewing technique is necessary. If water is too hot, it can cause scorching and off flavors in more delicate white and green teas, while excessive steeping times can cause accumulation of tannins and other bitter flavor compounds. Below are some recommended brewing times and temperatures for different tea types.

Tea type	Water temperature	Steeping time (loose leaf)	Steeping time (bag)
White tea	170–180 °F	1–3 minutes	30–60 seconds
Green tea	170–180 °F	3–4 minutes	1–3 minutes
Oolong tea	170–180 °F	3–5 minutes	3–5 minutes
Black tea	190–210 °F	3–5 minutes	3 minutes
Dark or Pu-her tea[a]	190–210 °F	3–5 minutes	N/A

[a] Most dark teas are purchased in compressed bricks and are not sold as tea bags

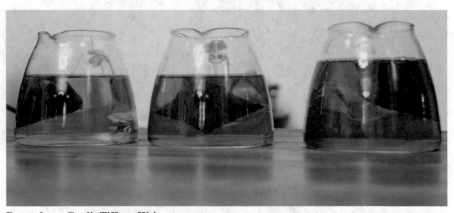

Brewed tea. Credit Tiffany Weir

References

Alemdaroglu, N.C., Dietz, U., Wolffram, S., Spahn-Langguth, H., & Langguth, P. (2008 Sep 1). Influence of green and black tea on folic acid pharmacokinetics in healthy volunteers: potential risk of diminished folic acid bioavailability. Biopharmaceutics & Drug Disposition [Internet]. [Cited 2021 Apr 12];29(6):335–48. Available from: http://doi.wiley.com/10.1002/bdd.617

Asbaghi, O., Fouladvand, F., Gonzalez, M. J., Aghamohammadi, V., Choghakhori, R., & Abbasnezhad, A. (2019). The effect of green tea on C-reactive protein and biomarkers of oxidative stress in patients with type 2 diabetes mellitus: a systematic review and meta-analysis. *Complementary Therapies in Medicine Churchill Livingstone, 46,* 210–216.

Banerjee, B. (1992). Botanical classification of tea. In *Tea.* [Internet]. Springer Netherlands. 1992 [cited 2021 Apr 15]. p. 25–51. Available from: https://link.springer.com/chapter/10.1007/978-94-011-2326-6_2

Chen, Y., Li, W., Qiu, S., Vladmir, C., Xu, X., Wang, X., et al. (2020 Feb 28). Tea consumption and risk of diabetes in the Chinese population: A multi-centre, cross-sectional study. *The British Journal of Nutrition.* [Internet]. [Cited 2021 Apr 15];123(4):428–36. Available from: https://doi.org/10.1017/S000711451900299X

Freeman, M., & Ahmed, S. (2011). *Tea horse road: China's ancient trade road to Tibet.* River Books Co, Ltd.

Fu, D., Ryan, E. P., Huang, J., Liu, Z., Weir, T. L., Snook, R. L., et al. (2011). Fermented Camellia sinensis, Fu Zhuan tea, regulates hyperlipidemia and transcription factors involved in lipid catabolism. *Food Research International, 44*(9).

Higginbotham, D., & Labaree, B. W. (1965 Jun 1). The Boston tea party. *Journal of American History.* [Internet]. [Cited 2021 Apr 12];52(1):114. Available from: https://academic.oup.com/jah/article-lookup/doi/10.2307/1901136

Hilary, J, & Dromey, J. (2010). A bitter cup [Internet]. Available from: https://waronwant.org/resources/bitter-cup

Huang J, Wang Y, Xie Z, Zhou Y, Zhang Y, & Wan X. (2014). *The anti-obesity effects of green tea in human intervention and basic molecular studies* [Internet]. Vol. 68, European Journal of Clinical Nutrition. Nature Publishing Group; [cited 2021 Apr 14]. pp. 1075–87. Available from: https://pubmed.ncbi.nlm.nih.gov/25074392/

Huang, F., Zheng, X., Ma, X., Jiang, R., Zhou, W., Zhou, S., et al. (2019 Dec 1). Theabrownin from Pu-erh tea attenuates hypercholesterolemia via modulation of gut microbiota and bile acid metabolism. *Nature Communications.* [Internet]. [Cited 2021 Apr 15];10(1):1–17. Available from: https://doi.org/10.1038/s41467-019-12896-x

Igho-Osagie, E., Cara, K., Wang, D., Yao, Q., Penkert, L.P., & Cassidy, A. et al. (2020 Dec 1). Short-Term Tea Consumption Is Not Associated with a Reduction in Blood Lipids or Pressure: A Systematic Review and Meta-Analysis of Randomized Controlled Trials. *Journal of Nutrition* [Internet]. [Cited 2021 Apr 14]; 150(12):3269–3279. Available from: https://academic.oup.com/jn/article/150/12/3269/5981794

Jensen, G. S., Beaman, J. L., He, Y., Guo, Z., & Sun, H. (2016). Reduction of body fat and improved lipid profile associated with daily consumption of a puer tea extract in a hyperlipidemic population: a randomized placebo-controlled trial. *Clinical Interventions in Aging.* [Internet]. Mar 24 [cited 2021 Apr 15];11:367–76. Available from: /pmc/articles/PMC4818050/.

Kc, Y., Parajuli, A., Khatri, B. B., & Shiwakoti, L. D. (2020). Phytochemicals and quality of green and black teas from different clones of tea plant. *Journal of Food Quality, 2020.*

Keller, A. C., Weir, T. L., Broeckling, C. D., & Ryan, E. P. (2013a). Antibacterial activity and phytochemical profile of fermented Camellia sinensis (fuzhuan tea). *FRIN.* [Internet]. [Cited 2021 Jan 25]; Available from: https://doi.org/10.1016/j.foodres.2013.04.023

Keller, A. C., Weir, T. L., Broeckling, C. D., & Ryan, E. P. (2013b). Antibacterial activity and phytochemical profile of fermented Camellia sinensis (fuzhuan tea). *Food Research International, 53*(2).

Ketchum, R. M. (2002). *Divided loyalties: how the American revolution came to New York.* [Internet]. Henry Holt & Co. [Cited 2021 Apr 12]. Available from: https://www.amazon.com/Divided-Loyalties-American-Revolution-Came/dp/0805061193

Kim, Y., Goodner, K. L., Park, J. D., Choi, J., & Talcott, S. T. (2011. 2011 Dec 15). Changes in antioxidant phytochemicals and volatile composition of Camellia sinensis by oxidation during tea fermentation. *Food Chemistry, 129*(4), 1331–1342.

Kitamura, S. (1950). On tea and camellias. *Acta Phytotaxonomica et Geobotanica.* 1950 Feb 28, *14*(2), 56–63.

Lin, Y. S., Tsai, Y. J., Tsay, J. S., & Lin, J. K. (2003). Factors affecting the levels of tea polyphenols and caffeine in tea leaves. *Journal of Agricultural and Food Chemistry, 51*(7), 1864–1873. 2003 Mar 26.

Lin, Y., Shi, D., Su, B., Wei, J., Găman, M., Sedanur Macit, M., et al. (2020 Oct 5). The effect of green tea supplementation on obesity: A systematic review and <scp>dose–response meta-analysis</scp> of randomized controlled trials. *Phyther Research* [Internet]. [Cited 2021 Apr 14]; 34(10), 2459–2470. Available from: https://onlinelibrary.wiley.com/doi/10.1002/ptr.6697

Lin, F.-J., Wei, X.-L., Liu, H.-Y., Li, H., Xia, Y., Wu, D.-T., et al. (2021). State-of-the-art review of dark tea: from chemistry to health benefits. *Trends Food Sci Technol [Internet], 109*, 126–138. Available from: https://doi.org/10.1016/j.tifs.2021.01.030

Liu, X., Xu, W., Cai, H., Gao, Y.-T., Li, H., Ji, B.-T., et al. (2018). Green tea consumption and risk of type 2 diabetes in Chinese adults: The Shanghai women's health study and the Shanghai men's health study. *International Journal of Epidemiology.* [Internet]. 2018 Dec 1 [cited 2021 Apr 15];47(6):1887–96. Available from: https://academic.oup.com/ije/article/47/6/1887/5086723

Long, J. (2014). Fairtrade and rainforest Alliance failing to deliver a living wage? *Ethical Consumer.* [Internet]. Available from: www.ethicalconsumer.org

Martin, L. C. (2007). *Tea: The drink that changed the world.* [Internet]. Tuttle Publishing. [Cited 2021 Apr 12]. Available from: https://www.abebooks.com/servlet/BookDetailsPL?bi=30869142740&searchurl=isbn%3D9780804837248%26sortby%3D17&cm_sp=snippet-_-srp1-_-title16

Nie, J., Yu, C., Guo, Y., Pei, P., Chen, L., Pang, Y., et al. (2021). Tea consumption and long-term risk of type 2 diabetes and diabetic complications: a cohort study of 0.5 million Chinese adults. *The American Journal of Clinical Nutrition.* [Internet]. 2021 Mar 11 [cited 2021 Apr 15]; Available from: https://academic.oup.com/ajcn/advance-article/doi/10.1093/ajcn/nqab006/6168524

Okakura, K. (1906). *The book of tea* (p. 160). Fox, Duffield & Company.

Ping, G. Z., Ouyang, J., Lan, W. X., Zhou, F., Lu, D. M., Zhao, C. J., et al. (2020. 2020 Oct 1). Dark tea extracts: chemical constituents and modulatory effect on gastrointestinal function. *Biomedicine & Pharmacotherapy, 130*, 110514.

Robins, N. (2006). *The corporation that changed the world.* [Internet]. Pluto Press. [Cited 2021 Apr 12]. Available from: https://www.plutobooks.com/9780745331959/the-corporation-that-changed-the-world/

Schwalfenberg, G., Genuis, S. J., & Rodushkin, I. (2013). The benefits and risks of consuming brewed tea: beware of toxic element contamination. *Journal of Toxicology, 2013*.

Shiraishi, M., Haruna, M., Matsuzaki, M., Ota, E., Murayama, R., & Murashima, S. (2010). Association between the serum folate levels and tea consumption during pregnancy. *Bioscience Trends, 4*(5), 225–230. 2010 Oct.

Somanchi, M., Phillips, K., Haile, E., & Pehrsson, P. Vitamin C content in dried and brewed green tea from the US retail market. The FASEB Journal [Internet]. [Cited 2021 Jan 19];31:956.8–956.8. Available from: https://faseb.onlinelibrary.wiley.com/doi/full/10.1096/fasebj.31.1_supplement.956.8

Takeda, R., Furuno, Y., Imai, S., Ide, Y., Wu, D., & Yan, K. (2019). Effect of powdered beverages containing Pu-erh tea extract on postprandial blood glucose levels. *Functional Foods in Health and Disease.* [Internet]. 2019 Aug 1 [cited 2021 Apr 15];9(8):532–42. Available from: https://www.ffhdj.com/index.php/ffhd/article/view/635/1001

Turner, J., & Webb, H. (2014). A Nice cup of tea. *Ethical Consumer.* [Internet]. Available from: www.ethicalconsumer.org

Webster, A. (2011). The twilight of the East India company: the evolution of Anglo-Asian commerce and politics, 1790–1860. *Victorian Studies, 54*(1), 125.

Weir, T., Hu, Y., Ryan, E., Fu, D., Xiao, W., Lin, W., Murray, P., & Snook, R. (2012). Medicinal Chinese teas: a review of their health benefits with a focus on fermented tea. *HerbalGram.* [Internet]. [Cited 2021 Apr 15];(94):42–7. Available from: https://www.herbalgram.org/resources/herbalgram/authors/weir-tiffany/

Xu, R., Yang, K., Ding, J., & Chen, G. (2020). *Effect of green tea supplementation on blood pressure: A systematic review and meta-analysis of randomized controlled trials* [Internet]. Vol. 99, Medicine (United States). Lippincott Williams and Wilkins; [cited 2021 Apr 14]. Available from: /pmc/articles/PMC7015560/

Yu, L., & Demi Hitz, F. R. C. (1974). *The classic of tea.* [Internet] Little Brown & Co. [Cited 2021 Apr 12]. Available from: https://www.amazon.com/Classic-Tea-Yu-Lu/dp/0316534501

Yu, J., Song, P., Perry, R., Penfold, C., & Cooper, A. R. (2017). The effectiveness of green tea or green tea extract on insulin resistance and Glycemic control in type 2 diabetes mellitus. *A Meta-Analysis.* [Cited 2021 Apr 14]; Available from: http://e-dmj.org

Zhang, C., Qin, Y. Y., Wei, X., Yu, F. F., Zhou, Y. H., & He, J. (2015). Tea consumption and risk of cardiovascular outcomes and total mortality: a systematic review and meta-analysis of prospective observational studies. *European Journal of Epidemiology.* [Internet] 2015 Mar 20 [cited 2021 Apr 14];30(2):103–13. Available from: https://pubmed.ncbi.nlm.nih.gov/25354990/

Zhong X, Zhang T, Liu Y, Wei X, Zhang X, Qin Y, et al. (2015). Short-term weight-centric effects of tea or tea extract in patients with metabolic syndrome: A meta-analysis of randomized controlled trials [Internet]. Vol. 5, Nutrition and Diabetes Nature Publishing Group [cited 2021 Apr 14]. p. e160–e160. Available from: www.nature.com/nutd

Chapter 12
Tree Berries

Rafaela G. Feresin, Rami S. Najjar, Maureen L. Meister,
and Jessica-Kim Danh

For centuries, civilizations across the world have utilized tree berry florae in various capacities from stimulating economic growth, improving agricultural practices, to improving health and nutrition. More recently, tree berry fruits have gained mainstream popularity through celebrity endorsements and are often referred to as a *superfood,* in part, due to their polyphenol content. Polyphenols are bioactive compounds produced exclusively in plants when they undergo stress (Manach et al., 2004). They are most known for their antioxidant capacity but have also been shown to have a wide range of beneficial health effects. This chapter will focus on açaí, amla, and mulberry, which are tree berries that possess great antioxidant capacity and health benefits.

12.1 Cultural History

12.1.1 *Açaí*

The Açaí berry is spherical and ripens to a dark purple when matured. It grows in açaí palm trees (*Euterpe oleracea* Mart) native to Central and South America and can be found growing in regions of the Amazon in both the swamps and plains. While açaí surged in popularity in North America after its promotion on the Oprah Winfrey show, its importance in its native region as an economic staple cannot be understated owing to its various uses not only as a food but also in food and cellulose production, animal feed, housing, and traditional medicine (Marcason, 2009).

R. G. Feresin (✉) · R. S. Najjar · M. L. Meister · J.-K. Danh
Georgia State University, Atlanta, GA, USA
e-mail: rferesin@gsu.edu

© The Author(s), under exclusive license to Springer Nature Switzerland AG 2022   157
J. P. Miller, C. Van Buiten (eds.), *Superfoods*, Food and Health,
https://doi.org/10.1007/978-3-030-93240-4_12

12.1.2   Amla

Amla (*Emblica officinalis* Gaertn or *Phyllanthus emblica* Linn), or Indian goose-berry, is one of the oldest fruits in India and is native across India, Sri Lanka, Malaysia, and China (Krishnaveni & Mirunalini, 2010). The fruits of Amla trees are spherical with a light-green coloring and smooth appearance and may be consumed raw or cooked into both sweet and savory dishes. The Amla tree is revered in Indian mythology as it is believed to be the first tree created in the universe (Kulkarni & Ghurghure, 2018). It is, perhaps, due to this hallowed position that Amla is used extensively in *Ayurveda* (an alternative system of medicine originating in India) in a potent group of drugs known as *rasayana*. Rasayana ingredients are believed to prevent aging and promote longevity (Kumar et al., 2012).

12.1.3   Mulberry

The Mulberry tree was domesticated thousands of years ago for its leaves, which were used to feed the larvae of silkworms in the practice of sericulture, the rearing of silkworms to produce silk (Chinnaswamy et al., 2012; Good, 2002). This long-standing practice dates back as early as the Yang-Shao Neolithic period (5000–3000 B.C.) in China and became an important industry during the nineteenth and early twentieth centuries in Europe, Japan, and Korea. This industry is now dominated by China and India (Good, 2002). There are over a thousand varieties of Mulberry under cultivation with additional uses in woodworking, landscaping, and medicine. Once matured, mulberry fruits may resemble blackberries in color or have a white to pink hue depending on the species. They can be enjoyed raw or processed into wine, juice, and jam. Folk medicine in China, Japan, and Korea have long included mulberry fruit as an ingredient for its pharmacological effects which include improvements in blood pressure, eyesight, and fever (Yuan & Zhao, 2017).

12.2   State of Nutrition Research

12.2.1   Açaí Berry

Much of the traditional applications of açaí palms have been shown to use all parts of the tree. For example, the stem and leaves have been used to relieve snake bites and muscular aches, the leaves have been used to alleviate chest pains, and the seeds have been processed into an oil to be consumed as an antidiarrheal agent (Yamaguchi et al., 2015). The berries themselves have become one of the most researched fruits recently following celebrity endorsements with much of the focus on its antioxidant activity (Yamaguchi et al., 2015). It should be noted that there are many claims that açaí berries may reduce weight, stop cancer, and even improve sexual performance; however, these claims are unsubstantiated.

Açaí is promoted for a high antioxidant content and health effects in combatting chronic disease. Açaí is a rich source of flavonoids including anthocyanins such as cyanidin-3-rutinoside, and flavones such as orientin, and hydroxybenzoic acids, including vanillic and syringic acids (Garzon et al., 2017; Schauss et al., 2006). Several clinical trials provide evidence that the consumption of açaí may indeed reduce oxidative stress, thus, potentially reducing the risk of chronic disease.

In obese subjects consuming a hypocaloric diet + 200 g frozen açaí daily for 90 days, a significant reduction in oxidative stress was observed (Aranha et al., 2020). Another study also indicates that daily consumption of 325 g of açaí pulp for 12 weeks reduces oxidative stress in obese men and women with metabolic syndrome, a cluster of metabolic risk factors (abdominal obesity, high blood pressure, high glucose levels, low high-density lipoprotein cholesterol (HDL-C), and high triglycerides) for cardiovascular diseases (Kim et al., 2018). Further, healthy human subjects consuming 200 mL/day of açaí showed increased serum total antioxidant capacity and antioxidant enzyme concentration compared to baseline (de Liz et al., 2020). These antioxidant effects are reflected clinically, as in a postprandial study in which healthy male subjects consumed 150 g açaí pulp in a smoothie with a high-fat meal, a significant improvement in vascular function was noted (Alqurashi et al., 2016).

These findings indicate that açaí may reduce cardiovascular disease risk due to a reduction in oxidative stress. These protective effects were observed with a single açaí-containing smoothie and with chronic açaí consumption across a spectrum of subjects: healthy and obese, as well as young and old. Protective effects were observed with 2/3 to 1 cup of açaí per day.

12.2.2 Amla

Amla has a ferric reducing antioxidant power (FRAP) score, a measure of antioxidant capacity, of ~261 mmol, which is exceptionally high compared to commonly consumed berries such as blackberries (~4 mmol), raspberries (~2.3 mmol), and blueberries (~1.9 mmol) (Carlsen et al., 2010). Amla contains several unique polyphenols such as mucic acid-1,4-lactone-3-O-gallate, hamamelitannin and isocorilagin (Li et al., 2019) and it is touted for its antidiabetic and cholesterol reducing effects demonstrated in a number of clinical studies (Akhtar et al., 2011; Antony et al., 2008; Kapoor et al., 2020; Upadya et al., 2019; Usharani et al., 2013, 2019; Jacob et al., 1988). For example, consumption of 1, 2, and 3 g of amla for 21 days reduced fasting and 2-h postprandial blood glucose levels in healthy and type 2 diabetic individuals (Akhtar et al., 2011). The same study also indicated that 1, 2, and 3 g of amla reduced fasting triglycerides, total cholesterol and increased HDL-C in type 2 diabetic patients while only 2 and 3 g elicited the same outcome in healthy individuals. All three doses of amla decreased low density lipoprotein cholesterol

(LDL-C) in healthy and type 2 diabetic individuals. Further, studies also demonstrated that daily consumption of 250 and 500 mg of amla powder for 12 weeks improved endothelial function and reduced serum markers of oxidative stress and inflammation in individuals with type 2 diabetes (Usharani et al., 2013) and metabolic syndrome (Usharani et al., 2019). Thus, amla is likely efficacious to reduce disease-risk in healthy individuals and improve risk factors in individuals with type 2 diabetes and metabolic syndrome.

12.2.3 Mulberry

Mulberry is one of the first fruits to be included as a medicinal-and-edible plant in the Chinese pharmacopoeia, as designated by the Ministry of Health of China in 1985. The British Pharmacopoeia lists Mulberry juice as an official drug as one of its uses in modern medicine is in the preparation of syrups such as those found in cough syrups (Venkatesh & Chauhan, 2008). Mulberry fruit has also been credited with having liver and kidney protective effects, relieving sore throat, and treating urinary incontinence, tinnitus, dizziness, constipation, and anemia (Venkatesh & Chauhan, 2008).

Mulberries have been publicized for their weight-lowering, cholesterol lowering and anti-diabetic effects. They are a rich source of polyphenols, particularly cyanidin-3-glucoside, quercetin, catechins and gallic acid (Yuan & Zhao, 2017). While human studies are scarce, limited preclinical evidence suggests anti-obesity, cardio-protective and anti-diabetic effects. Mulberries likely exert their cardio-protective effects by decreasing vascular oxidative stress and inflammation. For example, mulberry extract administered by oral gavage at a concentration of 200 and 300 mg/kg for 8 weeks reduced oxidative stress in old rats (Lee et al., 2020). Of note, oxidative stress was reduced in old rats to a level similar to young rats.

In addition, a 5 and 10% mulberry diet reduced oxidative stress and serum LDL-C in high-fat diet fed (HFD) rats (Yang et al., 2010). Further, in high-cholesterol-fed rabbits, a 0.5 and 1% mulberry diet dose-dependently reduced serum LDL-C and reduced atherosclerotic lesion severity induced by high-cholesterol feeding (Chen et al., 2005). Mulberries may directly inhibit the rate limiting enzyme in cholesterol metabolism, lending to these effects (Peng et al., 2011); thus, mulberries may function mechanistically as a statin. In several preclinical studies, mulberries appear to have anti-diabetic effects as well (Chang et al., 2013; Taghizadeh et al., 2017; Wang et al., 2013; Yan et al., 2016).

In a randomized, placebo-controlled trial, obese, middle-aged men and women with diabetic nephropathy consumed 300 mg/day of mulberry extract for 12 weeks (Taghizadeh et al., 2017). While subjects in both mulberry and placebo group did not lose weight, participants consuming mulberry extract had significantly reduced fasting blood glucose, triglycerides, and very-low density lipoprotein cholesterol (VLDL-C) compared to control. Further, high-sensitivity C-reactive protein (*hs*-CRP), a marker of systemic inflammation, as well as serum total antioxidant capacity and serum nitric oxide, a potent vasodilator, significantly improved in the mulberry group compared to placebo. While overall, animal studies in the treatment of cardiovascular disease, diabetes and obesity utilizing mulberry are compelling, there are only a limited number of investigations paired with a near absence of human studies. Thus, more research is needed to evaluate the protective effects of mulberries, with an emphasis on human studies.

12.3 Other Botanical and Chemical Properties

The rich nutritional benefits discussed above are unique to the berry of the tree and their polyphenolic profile in each instance. However, consideration should also be given to the other botanical portions of the plant including the leaves, bark and branches rich in protein and polysaccharides, which are known to have their own benefit. Extensive work continues to focus on identification and characterization of the active component in these berries and their other botanical components to extend their use.

Polysaccharide fractions extracted from açaí pulp, and not their polyphenol fractions, were responsible for the immunoregulatory properties, inciting neutrophil recruitment and T cell stimulation exhibiting a potential for use in the prophylactic treatment of infectious disease (Holderness et al., 2011). Similarly, açaí berry polysaccharide extracts enhanced clearance, and was more effective than other fruit derived polysaccharides, of a common pulmonary pathogen, suggesting possible use as a complement to antibiotic therapies against certain bacterium (Skyberg et al., 2012).

Ayurvedic healers claim that regular consumption of Amla will extend life beyond 100 years. The medical effects attributed to the use of Amla are wide-ranging from boosting immunity to treating respiratory disorders, diabetes, heart disease, rheumatism, and more (Kumar et al., 2012). In addition, evidence of the benefit of the polysaccharide fraction in amla has also been demonstrated (Li et al., 2018). Amla polysaccharides demonstrated potent antioxidant activity in a number of antioxidant assays (Li et al., 2018). Thus, every component of these superfood tree berries may be of benefit.

Mulberry is a multi-functional plant with highly palatable leaves. In addition to the widely consumed whole berry, white mulberry leaf powder has been suggested for use in the supplementation of nutrients in commercial food products (Srivastava et al., 2006). Additionally, mulberry leaf polysaccharide extracts are noted to have a multitude of bioactivities but most investigation has focused on the anti-diabetic effects including the potential to reduce fasting blood glucose levels and enhance insulin sensitivity (Cai et al., 2016; Jiao et al., 2017; Zhang et al., 2014). Further evidence has demonstrated the potent antioxidant activity of crude mulberry leaf polysaccharide *in vitro* (Yuan et al., 2015) suggesting antioxidant effects extending beyond the berry alone.

12.4 Social Issues

The growing demand for superfood products, specifically those generated from trees, has contributed to a shift in production considerations in areas where the indigenous communities had previously perfected production methods. The açaí berry is primarily cultivated in the Amazon basin. The rapid growth in popularity of the açaí berry in the early 2000s has contributed to significant changes in forest structure and the açaí palm that once promoted biodiversity in a non-timber forest farm, is becoming a detriment to the ecosystem. Recent increases in demand for the berry has led producers to increase production by increasing the density of the palms. This has led to significant thinning of other crops, contributing to homogenization of the plant community (Freitas et al., 2015) and a significant decline in avian diversity (Moegenburg & Levey, 2002). Aside from the harvesting of the açaí berry itself, other varieties, namely *Euterpe edulisi,* are being harvested for pulp, requiring complete destruction of the plant, and contributing the threat for extinction. To address major sustainability concerns, Sambazon, the leading exporter of the berry, has launched sustainable management efforts to protect the Amazon biodiversity and reduce risk to endangered species (Sambazon, n.d.). Continued efforts will need to be employed to sustain the açaí berry supply and protect the areas in which it is produced.

While the increase in demand of some superfoods, such as the açaí berry, has caused ecological difficulty, other superfoods and their plants may potentially serve as an environmental protectant. The white mulberry tree for example, primarily found in China, Japan and India, is used for its foliage in silkworm rearing, employed in the commercial production of silk and has been reviewed further for its ecological potential. While agricultural practices have focused exclusively on enhancing foliage production with the commercial production of mulberry trees for their fruit or leaves only being considered in the last few decades. As previously discussed, the mulberry fruit offers a significant nutritional benefit; however, as they are highly perishable and fragile, the price per pound ranges between U$10 and 15, creating an economical benefit for farmers but leaving their use and availability to consumers limited. More commonly sought after for use, with additional nutritional benefit, are the leaves of the mulberry tree. In addition to the use in human consumption as described, the incorporation of mulberry leaves into livestock feed has gained significant attention. The nutritional value of the mulberry leaf is 40–50% higher than other leguminous pasture and with high digestion rates, studies have shown benefit in milk-producing cow's output with reduced cost (Yupakarn et al., 2015).

In addition to the economic opportunity available in the use of the mulberry tree, it has also been recognized for its role in the prevention of ecological decline. The mulberry tree serves as deterrent against air pollutants with significant absorption capacity for sulfur dioxide, chloride, hydrogen fluoride and carbon (Jian et al., 2012). The mulberry tree is a carbon sink, absorbing approximately 135 kg of carbon annually and having high endurance specifically against sulfur (Jian et al., 2012). The mulberry root system has been shown to effectively reduce erosion rates of soil (Deepa et al., 2020) and reduce water run off rates while promoting soil enrichment (Rohela et al., 2020). As the mulberry tree is an environmentally adaptable plant with resistance to flood, draught, and air pollution, with positive attributes to the ecological and economical industries, the use of the mulberry tree in other industries should continue to be exploited.

Non-timber forest products, such as açaí described above and amla, often play an integral role in the social and economic status of local communities in which they are grown. Amla fruit is not only utilized for medicinal purposes, but it is also an important feeding preference for frugivores such as deer, bear, and antelope. Amla constitutes one of the most important forest products in southern India, meeting as much as 60% of the area's income (Ganesan & Siddappa Setty, 2003). Thus, preservation of amla fruit has major societal benefit for the indigenous population of India.

12.5   Recipe

Açaí Bowl
Servings: 1

Ingredients:

- 2 pack (8 oz) frozen açaí pulp
- ½ medium banana, frozen
- ½ cup of berries, frozen
- 1 tablespoon of honey

Suggested Toppings (to taste):

- Unsweetened coconut flakes
- Granola
- Banana, sliced
- Kiwi, sliced
- Berries

Instructions:

- Place all ingredients in a large blender. Blend on high until you reach a consistency of a thick smoothie.
- Sprinkle with toppings and enjoy!

Mulberry Sorbet (Yummly.com)
Servings: 4

Ingredients

- 3 cups of frozen black mulberries
- 1 tablespoon of honey
- 1 tablespoon of lemon juice

Instructions

- Pulse mulberries, honey, and lemon juice until soft
- Serve immediately or put in a plastic jar and refrigerate.

Amla Juice (Times of India)
Ingredients

- 8 medium amla, deseeded
- 1 tablespoon of honey
- ½ teaspoon of green cardamom
- water as needed
- 4 teaspoons of sugar
- ¼ teaspoon of salt
- ice cubes as needed

Instructions

- Grate or finely chop amla.
- Blend the grated or chopped amla with water until it turns into a fine paste. Strain it well.
- Add sugar, honey, cardamom, salt and blend it again.
- Pour the blended amla juice into a glass and serve with ice-cubes.

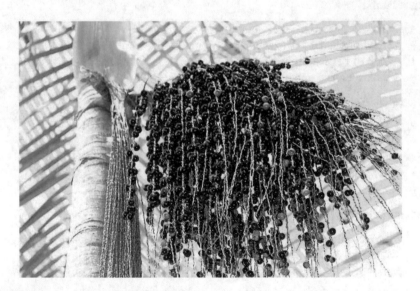

Ripe and unripe açaí berries on palm tree, Brazil
Credit: mspoli/iStock Photo

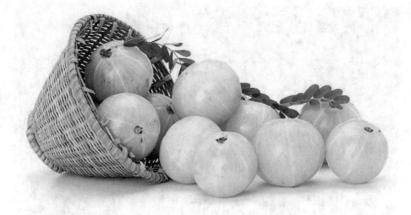

Amla (Indian Gooseberries)
Credit: Qpicimages/iStock Photo

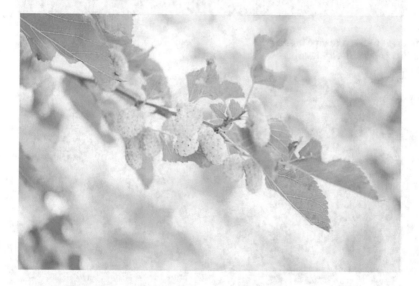

White Mulberry
Credit: Nastasic/iStock Photo

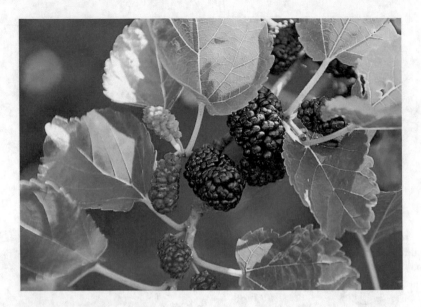

Black ripe and red unripe mulberries
Credit: syaber/iStock Photo

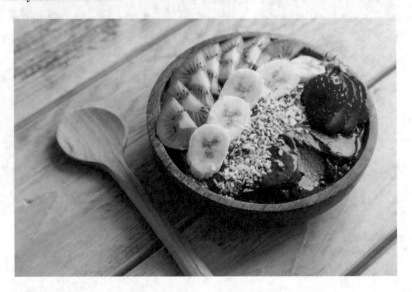

Açaí bowl with toppings
Credit: locknloadlabrador/iStock Photo

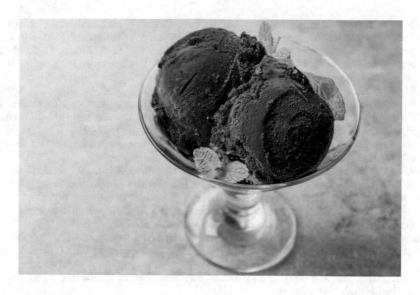

Mulberry Sorbet
Credit: alpaksoy/iStock Photo

References

Akhtar, M. S., Ramzan, A., Ali, A., & Ahmad, M. (2011). Effect of Amla fruit (Emblica officinalis Gaertn.) on blood glucose and lipid profile of normal subjects and type 2 diabetic patients. *International Journal of Food Sciences and Nutrition, 62*, 609–616.

Alqurashi, R. M., Galante, L. A., Rowland, I. R., Spencer, J. P., & Commane, D. M. (2016). Consumption of a flavonoid-rich acai meal is associated with acute improvements in vascular function and a reduction in total oxidative status in healthy overweight men. *The American Journal of Clinical Nutrition, 104*, 1227–1235.

Antony, B., Benny, M., & Kaimal, T. N. (2008). A pilot clinical study to evaluate the effect of Emblica officinalis extract (Amlamax) on markers of systemic inflammation and dyslipidemia. *Indian Journal of Clinical Biochemistry, 23*, 378–381.

Aranha, L. N., Silva, M. G., Uehara, S. K., Luiz, R. R., Nogueira Neto, J. F., Rosa, G., & Moraes De Oliveira, G. M. (2020). Effects of a hypoenergetic diet associated with acai (Euterpe oleracea Mart.) pulp consumption on antioxidant status, oxidative stress and inflammatory biomarkers in overweight, dyslipidemic individuals. *Clinical Nutrition, 39*, 1464–1469.

Cai, S., Sun, W., Fan, Y., Guo, X., Xu, G., Xu, T., Hou, Y., Zhao, B., Feng, X., & Liu, T. (2016). Effect of mulberry leaf (Folium Mori) on insulin resistance via IRS-1/PI3K/Glut-4 signalling pathway in type 2 diabetes mellitus rats. *Pharmaceutical Biology, 54*, 2685–2691.

Carlsen, M. H., Halvorsen, B. L., Holte, K., Bohn, S. K., Dragland, S., Sampson, L., Willey, C., Senoo, H., Umezono, Y., Sanada, C., Barikmo, I., Berhe, N., Willett, W. C., Phillips, K. M., Jacobs, D. R., Jr., & Blomhoff, R. (2010). The total antioxidant content of more than 3100 foods, beverages, spices, herbs and supplements used worldwide. *Nutrition Journal, 9*, 3.

Chang, J. J., Hsu, M. J., Huang, H. P., Chung, D. J., Chang, Y. C., & Wang, C. J. (2013). Mulberry anthocyanins inhibit oleic acid induced lipid accumulation by reduction of lipogenesis and promotion of hepatic lipid clearance. *Journal of Agricultural and Food Chemistry, 61*, 6069–6076.

Chen, C. L. L., Hsu, J., Huang, H., Yang, M., & Wang, C. (2005). Mulberry extract inhibits the development of atherosclerosis in cholesterol-fed rabbits. *Food Chemistry, 91*, 601–607.

Chinnaswamy, R., Lakshmi, H., Kumari, S. S., Anuradha, C. M., & Kumar, C. S. (2012). Nutrigenetic screening strains of the mulberry silkworm, Bombyx mori, for nutritional efficiency. *Journal of Insect Science, 12*, 3.

De Liz, S., Cardoso, A. L., Copetti, C. L. K., Hinnig, P. F., Vieira, F. G. K., Da Silva, E. L., Schulz, M., Fett, R., Micke, G. A., & Di Pietro, P. F. (2020). Acai (Euterpe oleracea Mart.) and jucara (Euterpe edulis Mart.) juices improved HDL-c levels and antioxidant defense of healthy adults in a 4-week randomized cross-over study. *Clinical Nutrition, 39*, 3629–3636.

Deepa, K. B., Vishaka, G. V., & Nithin Kumar, D. M. (2020). Mulberry as a avenue plant. *Journal of Pharmacognosy and Phytochemistry, 9*, 135–137.

Freitas, M. A. B., Vieira, I. C. G., Albernaz, A. L. K. M., Magalhaes, J. L. L., & Lees, A. C. (2015). Floristic impoverishment of Amazonian floodplain forests managed for acai fruit production. *Forest Ecology and Management, 351*, 20–27.

Ganesan, R., & Siddappa Setty, R. (2003). Regeneration of amla, an important non-timber forest product from southern India. *Conservation and Society, 2*, 365–375.

Garzon, G. A., Narvaez-Cuenca, C. E., Vincken, J. P., & Gruppen, H. (2017). Polyphenolic composition and antioxidant activity of acai (Euterpe oleracea Mart.) from Colombia. *Food Chemistry, 217*, 364–372.

Good, I. (2002). *The archaeology of early silk*. In Proceedings of the 8th Biennial Symposium of the Textile Society of America.

Holderness, J., Schepetkin, I. A., Freedman, B., Kirpotina, L. N., Quinn, M. T., Hedges, J. F., & Jutila, M. A. (2011). Polysaccharides isolated from acai fruit induce innate immune responses. *PLoS One, 6*, e17301.

Jacob, A., Pandey, M., Kapoor, S., & Saroja, R. (1988). Effect of the Indian gooseberry (amla) on serum cholesterol levels in men aged 35-55 years. *European Journal of Clinical Nutrition, 42*, 939–944.

Jian, Q., Ningjia, H., Yong, W., & Zhonghuai, X. (2012). Ecological issues of mulberry and sustainable development. *Journal of Resources and Ecology, 3*, 330–339.

Jiao, Y., Wang, X., Jiang, X., Kong, F., Wang, S., & Yan, C. (2017). Antidiabetic effects of Morus alba fruit polysaccharides on high-fat diet- and streptozotocin-induced type 2 diabetes in rats. *Journal of Ethnopharmacology, 199*, 119–127.

Kapoor, M. P., Suzuki, K., Derek, T., Ozeki, M., & Okubo, T. (2020). Clinical evaluation of Emblica Officinalis Gatertn (Amla) in healthy human subjects: Health benefits and safety results from a randomized, double-blind, crossover placebo-controlled study. *Contemporary Clinical Trials Communication, 17*, 100499.

Kim, H., Simbo, S. Y., Fang, C., Mcalister, L., Roque, A., Banerjee, N., Talcott, S. T., Zhao, H., Krezider, R. B., & Mertens-Talcott, S. U. (2018). Acai (Euterpe oleracea Mart.) beverage consumption improves biomarkers for inflammation but not glucose- or lipid-metabolism in individuals with metabolic syndrome in a randomized, double-blinded, placebo-controlled clinical trial. *Food & Function, 9*, 3097–3103.

Krishnaveni, M., & Mirunalini, S. (2010). Therapeutic potential of Phyllanthus emblica (amla): The ayurvedic wonder. *Journal of Basic and Clinical Physiology and Pharmacology, 21*, 93–105.

Kulkarni, K. V., & Ghurghure, S. M. (2018). Indian gooseberry (Emblica officinalis):Complete pharmacognosy review. *International Journal of Chemistry Studies, 2*, 05–11.

Kumar, K. S., Dutta, A., Yadav, A., Paswan, S., Srivastava, S., & Deb, L. (2012). Recent trends in potential traditional Indian herbs Emblica officinalis and its medicinal importance. *Journal of Pharmacognosy and Phytochemistry*, 24–32.

Lee, G. H., Hoang, T. H., Jung, E. S., Jung, S. J., HAN, S. K., Chung, M. J., Chae, S. W., & Chae, H. J. (2020). Anthocyanins attenuate endothelial dysfunction through regulation of uncoupling of nitric oxide synthase in aged rats. *Aging Cell, 19*, e13279.

Li, Y., Chen, J., Cao, L., Li, L., Wang, F., Liao, Z., Chen, J., Wu, S., & Zhang, L. (2018). Characterization of a novel polysaccharide isolated from Phyllanthus emblica L. and analysis of its antioxidant activities. *Journal of Food Science and Technology, 55*, 2758–2764.

Li, Y. Y., Guo, B. C., Wang, W. T., Li, L., Cao, L. L., Yang, C., Liu, J. Y., Liang, Q., Chen, J. J., Wu, S. H., & Zhang, L. Y. (2019). Characterization of phenolic compounds from Phyllanthus emblica fruits using HPLC-ESI-TOF-MS as affected by an optimized microwave-assisted extraction. *International Journal of Food Properties, 22*, 330–342.

Manach, C., Scalbert, A., Morand, C., Remesy, C., & Jimenez, L. (2004). Polyphenols: Food sources and bioavailability. *The American Journal of Clinical Nutrition, 79*(5), 727–747.

Marcason, W. (2009). What is the acai berry and are there health benefits? *Journal of the American Dietetic Association, 109*, 1968.

Moegenburg, S. M., & Levey, D. J. (2002). Prospects for conserving biodiversity in Amazonian extractive reserves. *Ecology Letters, 5*, 320–324.

Peng, C. H., Liu, L. K., Chuang, C. M., Chyau, C. C., Huang, C. N., & Wang, C. J. (2011). Mulberry water extracts possess an anti-obesity effect and ability to inhibit hepatic lipogenesis and promote lipolysis. *Journal of Agricultural and Food Chemistry, 59*, 2663–2671.

recipes.timesofindia.com. (n.d.). *Amla Juice Recipe: How to Make Amla Juice Recipe | Homemade Amla Juice Recipe.* [online] Available at: https://recipes.timesofindia.com/us/beverage/non-alcoholic/amla-juice/rs56167617.cms. Accessed 15 Jul. 2021.

Rohela, G. K., Muttanna, S. P., Kumar, R., & Chowdhury, S. R. (2020). Mulberry (Morus spp.): An ideal plant for sustainable development. *Trees, Forests and People, 2.*

Schauss, A. G., Wu, X., Prior, R. L., Ou, B., Patel, D., Huang, D., & Kababick, J. P. (2006). Phytochemical and nutrient composition of the freeze-dried amazonian palm berry, Euterpe oleraceae mart. (acai). *Journal of Agricultural and Food Chemistry, 54*, 8598–8603.

Skyberg, J. A., Rollins, M. F., Holderness, J. S., Marlenee, N. L., Schepetkin, I. A., Goodyear, A., Dow, S. W., Jutila, M. A., & Pascual, D. W. (2012). Nasal Acai polysaccharides potentiate innate immunity to protect against pulmonary Francisella tularensis and Burkholderia pseudomallei infections. *PLoS Pathogens, 8*, e1002587.

Srivastava, S., Kapoor, R., Thathola, A., & Srivastava, R. P. (2006). Nutritional quality of leaves of some genotypes of mulberry (Morus alba). *International Journal of Food Sciences and Nutrition, 57*, 305–313.

Taghizadeh, M., Soleimani, A., Bahmani, F., Moravveji, A., Asadi, A., Amirani, E., Farzin, N., Sharifi, N., Naseri, A., Dastorani, M., & Asemi, Z. (2017). Metabolic response to mulberry extract supplementation in patients with diabetic nephropathy: A randomized controlled trial. *Iranian Journal of Kidney Diseases, 11*, 438–446.

Upadya, H., Prabhu, S., Prasad, A., Subramanian, D., Gupta, S., & Goel, A. (2019). A randomized, double blind, placebo controlled, multicenter clinical trial to assess the efficacy and safety of Emblica officinalis extract in patients with dyslipidemia. *BMC Complementary and Alternative Medicine, 19*, 27.

Usharani, P., Fatima, N., & Muralidhar, N. (2013). Effects of Phyllanthus emblica extract on endothelial dysfunction and biomarkers of oxidative stress in patients with type 2 diabetes mellitus: A randomized, double-blind, controlled study. *Diabetes Metabolic Syndrome and Obesity, 6*, 275–284.

Usharani, P., Merugu, P. L., & Nutalapati, C. (2019). Evaluation of the effects of a standardized aqueous extract of Phyllanthus emblica fruits on endothelial dysfunction, oxidative stress, systemic inflammation and lipid profile in subjects with metabolic syndrome: A randomised, double blind, placebo controlled clinical study. *BMC Complementary and Alternative Medicine, 19*, 97.

Venkatesh, K. P., & Chauhan, S. (2008). Mulberry: Life enhancer. *Journal of Medicinal Plants Research, 2*, 271–278.

Wang, Y., Xiang, L., Wang, C., Tang, C., & He, X. (2013). Antidiabetic and antioxidant effects and phytochemicals of mulberry fruit (Morus alba L.) polyphenol enhanced extract. *PLoS One, 8*, e71144.

www.sambazon.com. (n.d.). *How to be a changemaker with our greenhouse initiative | Sambazon.* [online] Available at: https://www.sambazon.com/activism. Accessed 15 Jul 2021.

Yamaguchi, K. K., Pereira, L. F., Lamarao, C. V., Lima, E. S., & Da Veiga-Junior, V. F. (2015). Amazon acai: Chemistry and biological activities: A review. *Food Chemistry, 179*, 137–151.

Yan, F., Dai, G., & Zheng, X. (2016). Mulberry anthocyanin extract ameliorates insulin resistance by regulating PI3K/AKT pathway in HepG2 cells and db/db mice. *The Journal of Nutritional Biochemistry, 36*, 68–80.

Yang, X., Yang, L., & Zheng, H. (2010). Hypolipidemic and antioxidant effects of mulberry (Morus alba L.) fruit in hyperlipidaemia rats. *Food and Chemical Toxicology, 48*, 2374–2379.

Yuan, Q., & Zhao, L. (2017). The mulberry (Morus alba L.) fruit-A review of characteristic components and health benefits. *Journal of Agricultural and Food Chemistry, 65*, 10383–10394.

Yuan, Q., Xie, Y., Wang, W., Yan, Y., Ye, H., Jabbar, S., & Zeng, X. (2015). Extraction optimization, characterization and antioxidant activity in vitro of polysaccharides from mulberry (Morus alba L.) leaves. *Carbohydrate Polymers, 128*, 52–62.

Yupakarn, W., Lowilai, P., & Priprem, S. (2015). Effects of using Indian mulberry leaves as feed additives on feed digestion, ruminal fermentation and milk production in dairy cattle. *Pakistan Journal of Nutrition, 14*, 620–624.

Zhang, Y., Ren, C., Lu, G., Mu, Z., Cui, W., Gao, H., & Wang, Y. (2014). Anti-diabetic effect of mulberry leaf polysaccharide by inhibiting pancreatic islet cell apoptosis and ameliorating insulin secretory capacity in diabetic rats. *International Immunopharmacology, 22*, 248–257.

Chapter 13
Potatoes

Adam L. Heuberger, Janak R. Joshi, and Sahar Toulabi

13.1   The Cultural History of Potato

Roots and tubers have been central to the human diet for thousands of years. Roots and tubers are classified as vegetables and known for their excellent storage properties and density of macronutrients. Example roots include carrots, beets, parsnips, radishes, and sweet potatoes. While roots are mostly known as plant vegetative tissues that grow underground, some plant stems also exist beneath the soil. Examples include rhizome-based foods such as ginger, ginseng, and turmeric, but also starch-accumulating tissues known as tubers. From the plant's perspective, the purpose of these underground stems is to vegetatively spread to a new location to propagate, a clonal reproduction method that negates the need to flower and seed. Because these tissues are involved in reproduction, they ideally match macro- and micro-nutrient densities found in whole grains such as rice and wheat (e.g. starch, vitamins, minerals). But the fact that they grow underground means exposure to a wide range of stresses, and so plants also accumulate unique phytochemicals that mediate resistance to abiotic and biotic stresses. It is this reason that roots and tubers are somewhat unique, as they are vegetables with excellent nutrient and caloric density, but also contain phytochemicals that impact human health and disease, achieving the superfood status.

A. L. Heuberger (✉)
Department of Horticulture and Landscape Architecture, Colorado State University, Fort Collins, CO, USA

Department of Soil and Crop Sciences, Colorado State University, Fort Collins, CO, USA
e-mail: adam.heuberger@colostate.edu

J. R. Joshi · S. Toulabi
Department of Horticulture and Landscape Architecture, Colorado State University, Fort Collins, CO, USA

© The Author(s), under exclusive license to Springer Nature Switzerland AG 2022
J. P. Miller, C. Van Buiten (eds.), *Superfoods*, Food and Health,
https://doi.org/10.1007/978-3-030-93240-4_13

Potato (*Solanum tuberosum* L.) is a tuber and can be thought of as the most superior of the superfoods. While it is comparable to other roots and tubers in nutrient density, it has a dominant role in global nutrition and health. Today, it is the primary vegetable consumed worldwide and fourth most widely produced crop next to rice, maize, and wheat. The potato breeding and agronomic system has been optimized and currently provides the densest form of calories per area of cultivation.

This chapter will discuss why potato is indeed a superfood and is a model for understanding the value of roots and tubers in the food system. It has a fascinating history in its natural evolution and domestication by humans for agriculture, value in maintaining life for the human race, and has a unique chemistry directed by its life cycle and the corresponding value in nutrition and human disease.

13.1.1 Domestication and Distribution

The potato crop originates from modern-day Peru, however wild *Solanum* species have been reported in Argentina, Bolivia, and Mexico (Hijmans & Spooner, 2001). Potato was domesticated approximately 10,000 years ago in Southern Peru, from *Solanum brevicaule* via single domestication event (Spooner et al., 2005). Later, it was introduced to Africa and Europe in the sixteenth century CE following colonization and trade. Interestingly, potato was first grown in Europe for ornamental purposes (i.e. for its stunning flowers), until the mid-eighteenth century CE. Before this time, people feared poisoning by potato, as wild potatoes have phytochemicals that cause severe gastrointestinal discomfort, known as glycoalkaloids. Colonists also avoided consumption because it was not mentioned in religious texts, and underground stems were considered unnatural, an invention of the devil, gross, and bewildering. Despite these preconceptions, potatoes were given by Spanish colonists to their armies, and later found that sailors eating potatoes did not suffer from scurvy. This observation was a major discovery of nutritional value of potato for Europeans and shifted governments to encourage potato cultivation for food beyond South America.

Before potato was introduced into Europe, many countries were suffering famine. After its introduction, rural populations had access to a cheap bounty of nutrition that fueled a population boom through enhanced nutrition and public health. Eventually, the ability of the potato to grow in diverse topography and temperate climate made it a major food resource of Europe by 1800 CE. Later, it was introduced to China and East Asia to meet the food demand of increasing populations. Though potato was originated and domesticated in South America, it extended to North America in 1719 through trade. Currently, China and India are the two largest growers in the world.

Potato cultivation further impacted national economies by freeing other grains for export. The Spanish also used potato to feed slaves in silver mines, enabling large-scale mining which eventually resulted in a price revolution in Spain and elsewhere in Europe. Many there believe potato as a major enabler of European global colonization. The dependence of cultures on the potato is further demonstrated in the context of the 'Potato Famine', which was initiated by *Phytophthora infesans*, the agent of late-blight disease. In Ireland, the loss of potato farms in the context of a specific social, political, and economic structure played a key part in emigration of a people to many parts of the world. Altogether, potato has been closely associated with much of modern human history.

13.1.2 Potato in Global and U.S. Agriculture: Features of Modern-Day Production

Potato is a major food crop that is grown in over 100 countries. Potatoes are an inexpensive staple crop with the best nutritional values on a per-dollar basis compared to other raw vegetables, and they can be accessed year-round (USDA and NASS, 2020; Drewnowski & Rehm, 2013). The crop is used for variety of purposes, with less than 50% of tubers consumed fresh, and the rest are processed or reused as seed tubers. Overall, the global potato market is broken up into 3 segments: fresh, processed (frozen, dehydrated, chip), and seed potato. Of those, fresh produce has five main market classes: Round whites (chipping), Reds, Russets, Yellows, and Specialty. In 2019, worldwide potato production reached 371 million tons, which is the highest global production to date, with an annual increase rate of +3% from 2007 to 2019 and is expected to retain growth in years to come. However, frozen potato is the major processed product for use in fries, hash browns, mashed, battered/cooked, topped/stuffed, and others. The global frozen potato market is the highest growing sector with an expected compound annual growth rate of 3.8% from 2018 to 2025. Similarly, the seed potato market was valued near 17 billion USD in 2020 with projected compound annual growth rate of 0.8% during 2021–2026.

Seed certification is a formal seed system characterized by inspection of seed lot for its purity, quality, and disease incidence. The certification system is one of the major requirements for high yield with reduced risk to disease outbreaks. All potato parts are regulated for certification: seed tubers, true seeds, *in vitro* plantlets, microtubers, mini-tubers, and cuttings. However, the certification process varies depending on the producing and importing country/state/province. Certification tests are performed to issue a phytosanitary certificate that informs on variety, origin, and quarantine pathogens.

Potatoes are temperate crops and can be grown in places where soil temperature ranges between 4 and 30°C, with the ideal temperature ranging between 15 and 21°C. Because potatoes are nutrient-dense, the plants require a near-continuous supply of plant nutrients. The type and level of nutrient application (fertilization) depends on soil test results, variety planted, and crop rotation. Ideally, potato is best grown in fertile, well-drained soil that is rich in organic matter with a pH between 5.0 and 5.5. The recommended dose of fertilizer for potato is 165 kg/ha nitrogen; 145 kg/ha P_2O_5; 200 kg/ha K_2O. Potato fields are kept moist, but not fully wet nor dry. Wet fields will induce rotting of tubers, whereas dry field conditions will lead to cracked and knobby tubers. Overall, potato consumes 500–700 mm of water, from cultivation to harvest. Another important aspect of production is that the potato plant does not senesce naturally in some growing areas. In such fields, the potato plants is killed manually 10–25 days prior to harvesting to promote tuber maturation. This process is called haulm (vine) killing and it is also useful to reduce risk of disease infection and spread. Following production, tubers then undergo grading, which is one of the important post-harvest activities that results in the cleaning and sorting of consumable potatoes from wounded and infected tubers. The sorting activity also separates tubers into pools based on size which makes them easily marketable.

13.2 Survey of Current State of Nutritional Research

13.2.1 Overview of Potato Food Chemistry: Nutrients

As it exists today, most potato cultivars have adequate nutrition that lives up to its status as the world's most consumed vegetable. A 100 g serving of potato contains approximately 100 kcal comprised of 23% carbohydrate (starches and sugars), 2% protein, vitamins (B, E, K), more than 23 minerals (notably high potassium), and lipids (Table 13.1).

Potato starch is approximately 75% of the tuber mass (dry) and is a mixture of amylopectin and amylose. A consensus is to treat the resistant starch in potato tubers as 30% content, with a potential range between 20 and 40% (Jansen et al., 2001; Yusuph et al., 2003). Amylose starch is more likely to reach the colon where it can be fermented by commensal bacteria leading to short chain fatty acid production. A study of potato starch in rats showed effects on short chain fatty acid levels and the microbial composition of the cecum, notably increasing levels of butyrate and affecting fecal bile content (Han et al., 2008). In addition to starch, potato contains approximately 2 g of fiber, largely in the skin (Camire et al., 2009), and due to its high consumption, potato fiber is approximately 20% of the fiber consumed in the U.S. diet (Burgos et al., 2020). Other studies of potato starch find effects on reducing gut inflammation, reversing of microbial dysbiosis, gut brain signaling (Klingbeil et al., 2019), and no effects on blood glucose metabolism compared to controls, all while facilitating satiety (Sanders et al., 2021).

For protein, potato is considered low in content but high in quality. This is based on the composition of amino acids, closely resembling eggs, and considered to have better value than protein in rice, soybeans, and legumes. (Waglay & Karboune, 2016; Gorissen et al., 2018; Bártová et al., 2015; Bártová & Bárta, 2009). The main storage protein is patatin (40–60%), and is notable for having lipase activity and its ease of breaking down at rather low temperatures (~28 °C) (Pots et al., 1999). The primary effect of potato protein consumption is reduced overall food intake

Table 13.1 Estimated chemical content of one serving of potato

	per 100 g cooked potato tuber fresh weight[a]
Macronutrients	
Energy	100 kcal
Protein	2 g
Total lipids	0.1 g
Carbohydrates	23 g
Micronutrients	
Potassium	411 mg
Other minerals	147 mg
Vitamin C	15 mg
B vitamins	15 mg
Free amino acids	2.1 g
Bioactives[b]	
Phenolics (total)	1–400 mg
Phenolics (chlorogenic acids)	1–100 mg
Glycoalkaloids	1–20 mg
Polyamines	2–6 mg
Kukoamines	3.5 mg
Calystegines	0.34–6.8 mg
Carotenoids	10–310 mg
Anthocyanins	0.5–140 mg
Phytosterols	5 mg
Nitrates	1.5–50 mg

[a]Macro and micronutrients for fresh weight, USDA National Nutrient Database for Standard Reference (Release 28) for microwaved potato with skin
[b]Values are often reported uncooked; some values estimated based on 80% moisture conversion from reported dry weight values; phenolics/chlorogenic acid (Stushnoff et al., 2008; Friedman & Levin, 2009); anthocyanins in whole tuber fresh weight (skin and flesh) reported in (Jansen & Flamme, 2006); phytosterols and carotenoids (Piironen et al., 2003; Fernandez-Orozco et al., 2013); glycoalkaloids (Friedman & Levin, 2009; Kozukue et al., 2008; EFSA Panel on Contaminants in the Food Chain (CONTAM), 2020); calystegines (Friedman et al., 2003; Keiner & Dräger, 2000; Asano et al., 1997); kukoamines (Parr et al., 2005); nitrates (Lachman et al., 2005; Ierna, 2009); polyamines (Atiya Ali et al., 2011)

(Nakajima et al., 2011; Chen et al., 2012; Ku et al., 2016; Zhu et al., 2017). This is partially attributed to protease inhibitors (20–30% of potato protein), which have been isolated from potato and have been shown to affect satiety in rodent models and in people, leading to reduced food intake, and effects on gastrointestinal transit times and appetite hormone regulation (Flechtner-Mors et al., 2020; Komarnytsky et al., 2011). Therefore potato protein extracts are marketed as nutraceutical appetite suppressants. The protease inhibitor effect on may explain why as a so-called "starchy vegetable", tubers are more satiating than rice, wheat, and beans, with up to 40% less energy consumed with potato as the major starch in the diet (Flechtner-Mors et al., 2020; Johnston et al., 2020; Lee et al., 2019; Erdmann et al., 2007; Akilen et al., 2016; Geliebter et al., 2013). Further, isolated potato protein has other notable bioactive properties including antioxidant activity (Wu et al., 2020), they can prevent lipid oxidation (Wang & Xiong, 2005; Nieto et al., 2009; Cheng et al., 2010; Dastmalchi et al., 2016), can mediate DNA damage in cancer cell lines (Sun et al., 2013), have protective effects against ethanol-induced ulcers in mice (Kudo et al., 2009), and have inhibitory activity against angiotensin-converting enzyme (ACE) (Pihlanto et al., 2008; Mäkinen et al., 2016). Potato protein is also considered to have a low potential to form as an allergen (Waglay & Karboune, 2016).

Potato also contributes to global micronutrition (Nassar et al., 2012). Tubers are notably high in potassium, phosphorous, iron, zinc, B vitamins, and vitamin C. A study of consumption in the United Kingdom found that the proportion of micronutrients such as potassium, vitamin B6, vitamin C, fiber, folate, and magnesium was greater (9–15%) that the caloric contribution at 7% (Gibson & Kurilich, 2013).

13.2.2   Overview of Potato Food Chemistry: Bioactive Compounds

Further, as a vegetable, potato tuber contains common plant metabolites known to influence human health, specifically chlorogenic acid, flavonoids and other phenolics, phytosterols, kukoamines, biguanides, and bioactive proteins such as protease inhibitors, angiotensin converting enzyme inhibitors, and alpha-amylase inhibitors (Raigond et al., 2020). As protective metabolites for the plant, these compounds are often proportionally higher in the skin relative to the flesh. For yellow and orange fleshed cultivars, the predominant carotenoids are lutein and zeaxanthin (Breithaupt & Bamedi, 2002), and beta-carotene is typically a minor component. When evaluating food chemistry, it is critical to acknowledge that a potato tuber is living tissue, and its chemical composition will change during storage. For example, storage factors such as light, heat, temperature, and physical pressures (stacking/wounding) are known to affect the saccharide, glycoalkaloid, and calystegine content (Keiner & Dräger, 2000; Petersson et al., 2013; Kumar et al., 2004). While toxic, glycoalkaloids can be protective towards specific diseases, with anti-cancer, antimicrobial, and anti-inflammatory activity (Milner et al., 2011). The major phenolic, chlorogenic acid, has antioxidant, anti-inflammatory, neuroprotective, and effects towards cardiovascular disease, cancer, and diabetes (Naveed et al., 2018; Heitman & Ingram, 2017). Calystegines are potent glycosidase inhibitors with potential protection for diabetes (Jocković et al., 2013; Bourebaba et al., 2016). Kukoamines act as anti-cancer, anti-diabetes, neuroprotectants, and can reduce blood pressure (Wang et al., 2016; Zhao et al., 2020; Liu et al., 2017). The plant pigments carotenoids and anthocyanins act as antioxidants and facilitate cardiovascular health (Maria et al., 2015; Wallace et al., 2016).

13.2.3   Consumption of Whole Potato and Effects on Chronic Disease and Health

Despite the rich abundance of nutrients and bioactives in potato, some prospective cohort studies indicate negative health effects of including potato in the diet (Aune et al., 2017; Muraki et al., 2016) (Zhang et al., 2018). However, subsequent analyses clarified that most studies do not account for variation in processing methods, supporting that fried forms are the likely cause of negative health associations to potato (Aljuraiban et al., 2020). Similar results are not achieved when analyzing non-fried forms (boiled/baked/mashed), which were not associated with risk of obesity, diabetes, or cardiovascular disease (Schwingshackl et al., 2019; Attah et al., 2017; Borch et al., 2016). Animal models support a positive influence on health. For example, a mouse study that compared potato consumption relative to corn, wheat, and rice noted unique effects on short chain fatty acid producing gut microbes and microbiome analysis (gene abundances), supporting an influence on glycan metabolism and immune effects (Ruan et al., 2021). Effects of whole foods on cardiometabolic health include decreased serum lipid profiles in rats consuming a high-cholesterol diet (Han, 2013).

This evidence, that non-fried potato is beneficial, or at least not detrimental to health, was substantiated in a recent cross-over study that compared potato to refined grains. The study found that daily consumption of non-fried potato was linked to improved diet quality, and importantly did not exhibit an influence on blood glucose levels (Johnston et al., 2020). Several other reviews of observational studies indicate no or mild effects on disease risk factors with long-term consumption of whole potato (Moholdt et al., 2020; So et al., 2020). Increased satiety in adults and children has been observed following potato consumption (Erdmann et al., 2007; Akilen et al., 2016; Lee et al., 2020). Also related to lifestyle, potato was recently demonstrated as a sufficient fuel to sustain long-term exercise (Salvador et al., 2019). Further, beneficial cardiovascular effects have been described following consumption of whole potato, for example reduced oxidative stress, blood pressure, and arterial stiffness (Tsang et al., 2018; Vinson et al., 2012).

13.2.4   Anti-nutrition

While the tuber contains many compounds that promote health and act against disease, several compounds are noted to act adversely. While glycoalkaloids are toxic, this is dose-dependent, and a recent study support that there is no evidence of long-term adverse effects of glycoalkaloid consumption from Solanaceous plants (EFSA Panel on Contaminants in the Food Chain (CONTAM), 2020). While the phytosterol content of potato is considered low, these compounds do have the potential to form oxidized sterols during cooking. Similar to oxidized cholesterol, these oxyphytosterols can promote cardiovascular disease by increasing atheroscolerotic lesion formation (Brzeska et al., 2016; Plat et al., 2014). The other main anti-nutrient in potato is acrylamide, a cancer-promoting compound that forms when foods high in asparagine and glucose. Acrylamide occurs in potato chips and French fries at levels 10–100 fold higher compared to acrylamide found in bread and roasted nuts, and levels varied due to time of cooking and type of oil used for frying (Becalski et al., 2003).

13.2.5   The Challenge with Potato Food and Nutrition Research: There Is No One Potato

Whole food nutritional studies of potato are remarkably biased due to the differences in cultivar, agronomic, storage (the tuber is a living tissue), and processing conditions that all effect the chemistry of the finished food. As an example, one human study reported that pigmented (e.g. anthocyanin, carotenoid) whole potato consumption reduced markers of oxidative stress, however no effects were observed with non-pigmented potato (Kaspar et al., 2011). A rodent study reported similar differences, where inhibitory effects of breast cancer proliferation were stronger effects for pigmented varieties than a white potato (Thompson et al., 2009).

Other confounding factors are that tubers can be eaten with or without skin (which has a very distinct chemistry from the flesh), and nutrients and bioactives vary based on if they are boiled, baked, microwaved, or fried (Jayanty et al., 2019; Orsák et al., 2019; Furrer et al., 2018). The protein, glycoalkaloid, and nitrate content of the tuber largely differs among cultivars and growing conditions such as fertility (Lachman et al., 2005; Rogozińska et al., 2005; Mondy & Munshi, 1990). Vitamin C content reduces with cooking, but less so with microwaving compared to baking (Stushnoff et al., 2008). Minerals also vary among cultivars such as iron, zinc, and calcium (Nassar et al., 2012; Andre et al., 2007; Zhu et al., 2010; Deusser et al., 2012; Chaparro et al., 2018). The formation of acrylamide varies significantly based on potato variety and storage (25–2787 µg/kg), as the asparagine and carbohydrate content of the tubers are different (Mesias et al., 2018; Williams, 2005). It should also be noted that potato phenolics can mitigate the formation of acrylamide and the variation in varieties can affect content of the finished food (Zhu et al., 2010; Sordini et al., 2019; Qi et al., 2018), and phenolics can affect blood glucose metabolism (Moser et al., 2018).

13.3   Exploration of Related Science Topics

13.3.1   Other Aspects of Potato Plant Health that Impact Human Health

While much of a plant's chemistry is based on aspects of energy and reproductive biology, a second goal is to survive long enough to reach a reproductive state, which involves mechanisms of a plant response to external stresses. In the wild, potato tubers lay dormant through the winter at high altitudes, and the major chemical trait to withstand these conditions is through the production of suberin, the main chemical component of the skin. In potato, suberization occurs in response to tissue disruption, for example wounding. In development, this is a regular late-stage process by the tuber accumulates suberin on the exterior of tuber, maturing the skin near harvest. Suberin is a polymer of lipids crosslinked with glycerol and phenolics and is considered an insoluble fiber. Further, in plants, light stress is often mediated through light absorbing compounds such as anthocyanins and carotenoids. Like carrots, beets, and many other underground foods, potato tubers can accumulate anthocyanins and carotenoids in tubers, appearing as red, yellow/orange (very mild to very dark), or purple hues in the flesh and/or skin.

To manage pathogens, the tuber accumulates phytochemicals that are toxic or reduce fitness to microorganisms and pests. Following external fortifications of cell walls and skins, the main internal defense is through glycoalkaloids, compounds common to the Solanaceae plant family (e.g. tomato, eggplant, bell pepper), but mostly for green tissues. Through thousands of years of breeding, potatoes have been bred for low glycoalkaloids in the edible tissues, although exposing tubers to light will cause "greening" and subsequently high levels of these toxins. Other potato alkaloids that provide defense within the tubers are the kukoamines (phenolic polyamine alkaloids) and calystegines (tropane alkaloids), also common to the Solanaceae.

13.3.2   Evolution of S. tuberosum and Final Chemical Traits of the Potato Tuber

The evolution of S. tuberosum and subsequent domestication progressively shifted tubers into the chemistry of the food we know today. Approximately 200 wild species have been identified from South, Central, and North America (Hijmans & Spooner, 2001). An analysis of four wild potatoes revealed more than 50 variants of glycoalkaloids (Shakya & Navarre, 2008), and the final glycoalkaloid composition in domesticated potato is much lower and simpler (Chaparro et al., 2018). A genomic study on the evolution and domestication of potato supports selection of plant physiology (photoperiod, tuber cell cycle traits, reproduction), and an effect on glycoalkaloid biosynthesis, carbohydrate metabolism, and phenolics biosynthesis (Hardigan et al., 2017). Overall, the major effects of domestication trend towards increased tuber size and a decrease in the protective alkaloids toxic to humans (Kozukue et al., 2008). For starch, domestication shifted potatoes towards higher amylopectin/amylose ratios, only slightly higher starch yield, but notably higher granule particle size (Jansen et al., 2001).

13.4 Societal Issues of Potato

13.4.1 Sustainability and Environmental Health

As a vital global food crop, it is important to evaluate the potential for sustainable agricultural practices. Potato requires significant inputs in water and nitrogen, and phosphorous, as well as chemical inputs to combat fungi and nematodes. Scientists acknowledge the need for more sustainable potato production (Birch et al., 2012; Davenport et al., 2005; Ruark et al., 2014), and the industry has developed with significant technologies that enable precision agriculture (Cambouris et al., 2014; Alva et al., 2011). Recently, a study in China supports potato production as an environmentally responsible way of diversifying land used for the staple foods rice and wheat (Gao et al., 2019). Although it should be noted that the seed growing, certification, production, and storage components of the potato industry are resource intensive.

13.4.2 Current and Future Markets and Technologies

In addition to moving towards more sustainable management practices, the industry has the potential to bring greater diversity of cultivars to new markets. In general, there is low diversity available compared to the potential nutrient and bioactive content that can be achieved in a single tuber. Through breeding, it is possible to combine high carotenoid lines (yellow flesh) with anthocyanins (purple skins), with elevated levels of resistant starch and other nutrients. The specific genetic combinations, agronomic, storage, and processing practices have yet to be integrated to boost the maximum nutritional content available in this food. And so, while this chapter explores potato as a SuperFood, there is significant potential to continue to improve its impact on promoting human health and preventing disease. Several biofortification efforts are underway in potato, for example with zinc, iron, and iron availability (White et al., 2017; Andre et al., 2015). Further, as more is learned about the effects of potato bioactives, there is the potential to develop nutraceuticals originating from potato tuber, such as protein used as meat substitutes.

Other areas of change include shifting breeding to a new system. Potato production is largely clonal because of its tetraploid genetics and ease of vegetative reproduction. Recent efforts in breeding with diploid genetics are promising, and support the potential to match yield obtained in tetraploids, with the potential to achieve a hybrid system that can more easily incorporate novel traits from wild *Solanum* species (Jansky et al., 2016). There are also intense efforts in germplasm conservation within nationalities, in the public domain, and at international gene banks. The last area to explore is in genetic engineering, which is in practice but makes up a small portion of the market. Several studies report the potential for genetic engineering to enhance the nutritional quality of the tuber such as with increased beta-carotene (Van Eck et al., 2007), amylose (Zhao et al., 2018), and reduced acrylamide and browning (Waltz, 2015).

13.5   Recipes

Zesty Fingerling Potatoes
1 lb. fingerling potatoes, sliced in half lengthwise
1 heaping teaspoon sea salt or kosher salt
@1/2 tsp. fresh ground black pepper
½ tsp. ground oregano
Pinch of cayenne pepper
As needed – olive oil to coat generously
(optional – ¼ teaspoon finely chopped lemon zest or lemon peel)

Preheat oven to 400F.
Place the halved potatoes in a large mixing bowl with the remaining ingredients. Mix until the potatoes are well coated with oil and the other ingredients are well incorporated.
Spread the potatoes out on a baking sheet with a rim. Bake until tender and browned. Start checking for doneness after about 30 min. Serve immediately.
Recipe by Jeff Miller – used by permission.

Easy Yogurt Garlic Mashers
1 pound russet potatoes, cut into small cubes [peeling is optional]
½ tsp. salt
1 teaspoon garlic powder
½ cup Greek yogurt
¼ cup minced herbs as desired [chives are great, but your favorite herb works just as well]
To taste black pepper

Put the potatoes in a large pot. Cover with cold water. Bring to a boil and add the salt. Boil under tender.
Drain the potatoes. Put them back in the pot and mash them with the garlic powder.

Stir in the yogurt (and herbs if you are using them) and combine. Check the flavor and add more garlic powder, salt, or black pepper to season them to your taste. You can use more yogurt if the potatoes need more moisture.

Recipe by Jeff Miller – used by permission.

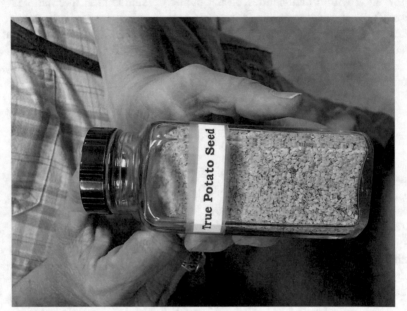

Photo by Sahar Toulabi – used by permission

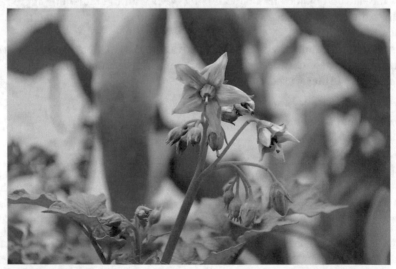

Samsmachado, CC BY 4.0 <https://creativecommons.org/licenses/by/4.0>, via Wikimedia Commons

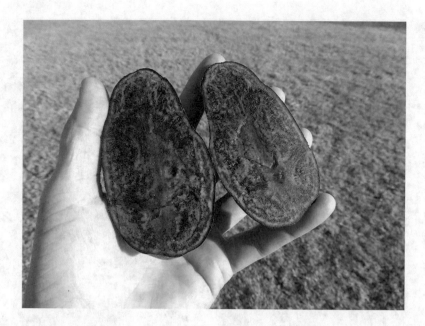

Forest & Kim Starr, CC BY 3.0 US <https://creativecommons.org/licenses/by/3.0/us/deed.en>, via Wikimedia Commons

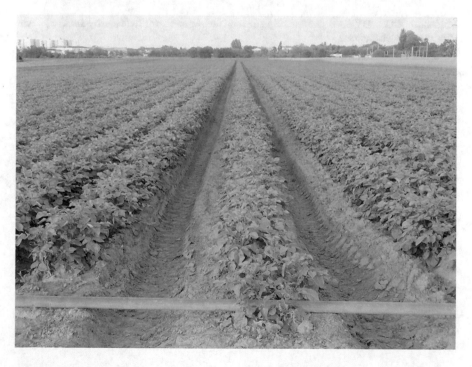

Sciencia58, CC BY-SA 4.0 <https://creativecommons.org/licenses/by-sa/4.0>, via Wikimedia Commons

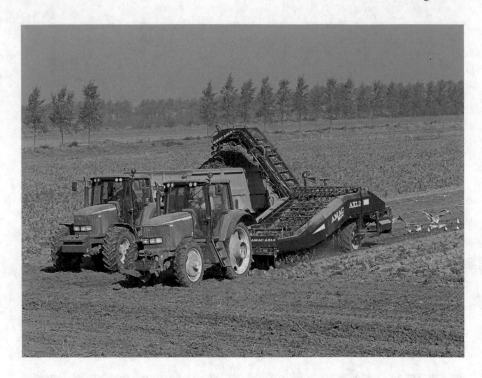

Rasbak, CC BY-SA 3.0 <https://creativecommons.org/licenses/by-sa/3.0>, via Wikimedia Commons

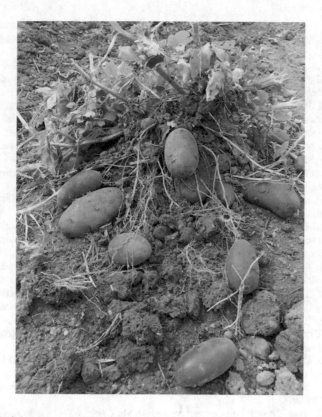

Freshly dug potatoes

References

Akilen, R., et al. (2016). The effects of potatoes and other carbohydrate side dishes consumed with meat on food intake, glycemia and satiety response in children, *Nutrition & Diabetes* 6(2), e195.

Aljuraiban, G. S., et al. (2020). Potato consumption, by preparation method and meal quality, with blood pressure and body mass index: The INTERMAP study, *Clinical Nutrition, 39*(10), 3042–3048.

Alva, A., et al. (2011). Improving nutrient-use efficiency in Chinese potato production: experiences from the United States, *Journal of Crop Improvement, 25*(1), 46–85.

Andre, C. M., et al. (2007). Andean potato cultivars (Solanum tuberosum L.) as a source of antioxidant and mineral micronutrients. *Journal of Agricultural and Food Chemistry, 55*(2), 366–378.

Andre, C. M., et al. (2015). In vitro bioaccessibility and bioavailability of iron from potatoes with varying vitamin C, carotenoid, and phenolic concentrations, *Journal of Agricultural and Food Chemistry, 63*(41), 9012–9021.

Asano, N., et al. (1997). The effects of calystegines isolated from edible fruits and vegetables on mammalian liver glycosidases, *Glycobiology, 7*(8), 1085–1088.

Atiya Ali, M., et al. (2011). Polyamines in foods: development of a food database, *Food & Nutrition Research, 55*(1), 5572.

Attah, A. O., Braaten, T., & Skeie, G. (2017). Change in potato consumption among Norwegian women 1998-2005-The Norwegian Women and Cancer study (NOWAC). *PloS One, 12*(6), e0179441.

Aune, D., et al. (2017). Fruit and vegetable intake and the risk of cardiovascular disease, total cancer and all-cause mortality—A systematic review and dose-response meta-analysis of prospective studies, *International Journal of Epidemiology, 46*(3), 1029–1056.

Bártová, V., & Bárta, J. (2009). Chemical composition and nutritional value of protein concentrates isolated from potato (Solanum tuberosum L.) fruit juice by precipitation with ethanol or ferric chloride, *Journal of Agricultural and Food Chemistry, 57*(19), 9028–9034.

Bártová, V., et al. (2015). Amino acid composition and nutritional value of four cultivated South American potato species. *Journal of Food Composition and Analysis, 40*, 78–85.

Becalski, A., et al. (2003). Acrylamide in foods: Occurrence, sources, and modeling, *Journal of Agricultural and Food Chemistry 51*(3), 802–808.

Birch, P. R., et al. (2012). Crops that feed the world 8: potato: Are the trends of increased global production sustainable?, *Food Security, 4*(4), 477–508.

Borch, D., et al. (2016). Potatoes and risk of obesity, type 2 diabetes, and cardiovascular disease in apparently healthy adults: A systematic review of clinical intervention and observational studies. *American Journal of Clinical Nutrition, 104*(2), 489–498.

Bourebaba, L., et al. (2016). Evaluation of antidiabetic effect of total calystegines extracted from Hyoscyamus albus, *Biomedicine & Pharmacotherapy, 82*, 337–344.

Breithaupt, D. E., & Bamedi, A. (2002). Carotenoids and carotenoid esters in potatoes (Solanum tuberosum L.): New insights into an ancient vegetable. *Journal of Agricultural and Food Chemistry, 50*(24), 7175–7181.

Brzeska, M., Szymczyk, K., & Szterk, A. (2016). Current knowledge about oxysterols: A review, *Journal of Food Science, 81*(10), R2299–R2308.

Burgos, G., et al. (2020). The potato and its contribution to the human diet and health. In *The Potato Crop* (pp. 37–74). Springer.

Cambouris, A. N., et al. (2014). Precision agriculture in potato production, *Potato Research, 57*(3–4), 249–262.

Camire, M. E., et al. (2009). Potatoes and human health, *Critical Reviews in Food Science and Nutrition, 49*(10), 823–840.

Chaparro, J. M., et al. (2018). Metabolomics and ionomics of potato tuber reveals an influence of cultivar and market class on human nutrients and bioactive compounds. *Frontiers in Nutrition, 5*(36).

Chen, W., et al. (2012). Suppressive effect on food intake of a potato extract (potein®) involving cholecystokinin release in rats. *Bioscience, Biotechnology, and Biochemistry, 76*(6), 1104–1109.

Cheng, Y., Xiong, Y. L., & Chen, J. (2010). Antioxidant and emulsifying properties of potato protein hydrolysate in soybean oil-in-water emulsions. *Food Chemistry, 120*(1), 101–108.

Dastmalchi, K., Wang, I., & Stark, R. E. (2016). Potato wound-healing tissues: A rich source of natural antioxidant molecules with potential for food preservation. *Food Chemistry, 210*, 473–480.

Davenport, J. R., et al. (2005). Environmental impacts of potato nutrient management, *American Journal of Potato Research, 82*(4), 321–328.

Deusser, H., et al. (2012). Polyphenol and glycoalkaloid contents in potato cultivars grown in Luxembourg. *Food Chemistry, 135*(4), 2814–2824.

Drewnowski, A., & Rehm, C. D. (2013). Vegetable cost metrics show that potatoes and beans provide most nutrients per penny. *PLoS One, 8*(5), e63277.

EFSA Panel on Contaminants in the Food Chain (CONTAM), et al. (2020). Risk assessment of glycoalkaloids in feed and food, in particular in potatoes and potato-derived products, *EFSA Journal,18*(8), e06222.

Erdmann, J., et al. (2007). Food intake and plasma ghrelin response during potato-, rice- and pasta-rich test meals. *European Journal of Nutrition, 46*(4), 196–203.

Fernandez-Orozco, R., Gallardo-Guerrero, L., & Hornero-Méndez, D. (2013). Carotenoid profiling in tubers of different potato (Solanum sp.) cultivars: Accumulation of carotenoids mediated by xanthophyll esterification, *Food Chemistry, 141*(3), 2864–2872.

Flechtner-Mors, M., et al. (2020). The effect of potato protease inhibitor II on gastrointestinal hormones and satiety in humans during weight reduction. *Diabetes, Metabolic Syndrome and Obesity: Targets and Therapy, 13*, 521–534.

Friedman, M., & Levin, C. E. (2009). Analysis and biological activities of potato glycoalkaloids, calystegine alkaloids, phenolic compounds, and anthocyanins. In *Advances in potato chemistry and technology* (pp. 127–161). Elsevier.

Friedman, M., et al. (2003). Glycoalkaloid and calystegine contents of eight potato cultivars, *Journal of Agricultural and Food Chemistry. 51*(10), 2964–2973.

Furrer, A. N., et al. (2018). Impact of potato processing on nutrients, phytochemicals, and human health, *Critical Reviews in Food Science and Nutrition, 58*(1), 146–168.

Gao, B., et al. (2019). Comprehensive environmental assessment of potato as staple food policy in China, *International Journal of Environmental Research and Public Health, 16*(15), 2700.

Geliebter, A., et al. (2013). Satiety following intake of potatoes and other carbohydrate test meals. *Annals of Nutrition & Metabolism, 62*(1), 37–43.

Gibson, S., & Kurilich, A. C. (2013). The nutritional value of potatoes and potato products in the UK diet, *Nutrition Bulletin, 38*(4), 389–399.

Gorissen, S. H. M., et al. (2018). Protein content and amino acid composition of commercially available plant-based protein isolates. *Amino Acids, 50*(12), 1685–1695.

Han, K. -H., et al. (2008). Feeding potato flakes affects cecal short-chain fatty acids, microflora and fecal bile acids in rats, *Annals of Nutrition and Metabolism, 52*(1), 1–7.

Han, K. -H., et al. (2013). Purple potato flake reduces serum lipid profile in rats fed a cholesterol-rich diet, *Journal of Functional Foods, 5*(2), 974–980.

Hardigan, M. A., et al. (2017). Genome diversity of tuber-bearing Solanum uncovers complex evolutionary history and targets of domestication in the cultivated potato, *Proceedings of the National Academy of Sciences,114*(46), E9999–E10008.

Heitman, E., & Ingram, D. K. (2017). Cognitive and neuroprotective effects of chlorogenic acid, *Nutritional Neuroscience, 20*(1), 32–39.

Hijmans, R. J., & Spooner, D. M. (2001). Geographic distribution of wild potato species. *American Journal of Botany, 88*(11), 2101–2112.

Ierna, A. (2009). Influence of harvest date on nitrate contents of three potato varieties for off-season production, *Food Composition and Analysis, 22*(6), 551–555.

Jansen, G., & Flamme, W. (2006). Coloured potatoes (Solanum tuberosum L.)–anthocyanin content and tuber quality. *Genetic Resources and Crop Evolution, 53*(7), 1321–1331.

Jansen, G., et al. (2001). Tuber and starch quality of wild and cultivated potato species and cultivars, *Potato Research, 44*(2), 137–146.

Jansky, S. H., et al. (2016). Reinventing potato as a diploid inbred line–based crop, *56*(4), 1412–1422.

Jayanty, S. S., Diganta, K., & Raven, B. (2019). Effects of cooking methods on nutritional content in potato tubers, *American Journal of Potato Research 96*(2), 183–194.

Jocković, N. A., et al. (2013). Inhibition of human intestinal α-glucosidases by calystegines, *Journal of Agricultural and Food Chemistry, 61*(23), 5550–5557.

Johnston, E. A., Petersen, K. S., & Kris-Etherton, P. M. (2020). Daily intake of non-fried potato does not affect markers of glycaemia and is associated with better diet quality compared with refined grains: A randomised, crossover study in healthy adults. *British Journal of Nutrition, 123*(9), 1032–1042.

Kaspar, K. L., et al. (2011). Pigmented potato consumption alters oxidative stress and inflammatory damage in men, *The Journal of Nutrition, 141*(1), 108–111.

Keiner, R., & Dräger, B. (2000). Calystegine distribution in potato (Solanum tuberosum) tubers and plants, *Plant Science,150*(2), 171–179.

Klingbeil, E. A., et al. (2019). Potato-resistant starch supplementation improves microbiota dysbiosis, inflammation, and gut–brain signaling in high fat-fed rats, *Nutrients, 11*(11), 2710.

Komarnytsky, S., Cook, A., & Raskin, I. (2011). Potato protease inhibitors inhibit food intake and increase circulating cholecystokinin levels by a trypsin-dependent mechanism. *International Journal of Obesity, 35*(2), 236–243.

Kozukue, N., et al. (2008). Distribution of glycoalkaloids in potato tubers of 59 accessions of two wild and five cultivated Solanum species, *Journal of Agricultural and Food Chemistry, 56*(24), 11920–11928.

Ku, S. K., et al. (2016). Anti-obesity and anti-diabetic effects of a standardized potato extract in Ob/Ob mice. *Experimental and Therapeutic Medicine, 12*(1), 354–364.

Kudo, K., et al. (2009). Antioxidative activities of some peptides isolated from hydrolyzed potato protein extract. *Journal of Functional Foods, 1*(2), 170–176.

Kumar, D., Singh, B. P., & Kumar, P. (2004). An overview of the factors affecting sugar content of potatoes. *Annals of Applied Biology, 145*(3), 247–256.

Lachman, J., et al. (2005). The effect of selected factors on the content of protein and nitrates in potato tubers, *Plant Soil and Environment, 51*(10), 431.

Lee, J. J., et al. (2019). Effect of potatoes and other carbohydrate-containing foods on cognitive performance, glycemic response, and satiety in children. *Applied Physiology Nutrition and Metabolism, 44*(9), 1012–1019.

Lee, J. J., et al. (2020). Effects of white potatoes consumed with eggs on satiety, food intake, and glycemic response in children and adolescents, *Journal of the American College of Nutrition, 39*(2), 147–154.

Liu, J., et al. (2017). Neuroprotective effects of Kukoamine A against cerebral ischemia via antioxidant and inactivation of apoptosis pathway, *Neurochemistry International, 107*, 191–197.

Mäkinen, S., et al. (2016). Angiotensin I-converting enzyme inhibitory and antihypertensive properties of potato and rapeseed protein-derived peptides. *Journal of Functional Foods, 25*, 160–173.

Maria, A. G., et al. (2015). Carotenoids: Potential allies of cardiovascular health?, *Food & Nutrition Research, 59*(1), 26762.

Mesias, M., et al. (2018). Acrylamide content in French fries prepared in households: A pilot study in Spanish homes. *Food Chemistry, 260*, 44–52.

Milner, S. E., et al. (2011). Bioactivities of glycoalkaloids and their aglycones from Solanum species, *Journal of Agricultural and Food Chemistry59*(8), 3454–3484.

Moholdt, T., Devlin, B. L., & Nilsen, T. I. L. (2020). Intake of boiled potato in relation to cardiovascular disease risk factors in a large Norwegian Cohort: The HUNT study, *Nutrients, 12*(1), 73.

Mondy, N. I., & Munshi, C. B. (1990). Effect of nitrogen fertilization on glycoalkaloid and nitrate content of potatoes, *Journal of Agricultural and Food Chemistry 38*(2), 565–567.

Moser, S., et al. (2018). Potato phenolics impact starch digestion and glucose transport in model systems but translation to phenolic rich potato chips results in only modest modification of glycemic response in humans, *Nutrition Research, 52*, 57–70.

Muraki, I., et al. (2016). Potato consumption and risk of type 2 diabetes: Results from three prospective cohort studies. *Diabetes Care, 39*(3), 376–384.

Nakajima, S., et al. (2011). Potato extract (potein) suppresses food intake in rats through inhibition of luminal trypsin activity and direct stimulation of cholecystokinin secretion from enteroendocrine cells. *Journal of Agricultural and Food Chemistry, 59*(17), 9491–9496.

Nassar, A. M., et al. (2012). Some Canadian-grown potato cultivars contribute to a substantial content of essential dietary minerals, *Journal of Agricultural and Food Chemistry, 60*(18), 4688–4696.

Naveed, M., et al. (2018). Chlorogenic acid (CGA): A pharmacological review and call for further research, *Biomedicine & Pharmacotherapy, 97*, 67–74.

Nieto, G., et al. (2009). Antioxidant and emulsifying properties of alcalase-hydrolyzed potato proteins in meat emulsions with different fat concentrations. *Meat Science, 83*(1), 24–30.

Orsák, M., et al. (2019). Chlorogenic acid content in potato tubers with colored flesh as affected by a genotype, location and long-term storage, *Plant, Soil and Environment, 65*(7), 355–360.

Parr, A. J., et al. (2005). Dihydrocaffeoyl polyamines (kukoamine and allies) in potato (Solanum tuberosum) tubers detected during metabolite profiling, *Journal of Agricultural and Food Chemistry, 53,* (13), 5461–5466.

Petersson, E. V., et al. (2013). Glycoalkaloid and calystegine levels in table potato cultivars subjected to wounding, light, and heat treatments, *Journal of Agricultural and Food Chemistry, 61*(24), 5893–5902.

Pihlanto, A., Akkanen, S., & Korhonen, H. J. (2008). ACE-inhibitory and antioxidant properties of potato (Solanum tuberosum). *Food Chemistry, 109*(1), 104–112.

Piironen, V., et al. (2003). Plant sterols in vegetables, fruits and berries, *Journal of the Science of Food and Agriculture, 83*(4), 330–337.

Plat, J., et al. (2014). Oxidised plant sterols as well as oxycholesterol increase the proportion of severe atherosclerotic lesions in female LDL receptor+/− mice, *British Journal of Nutrition, 111*(1), 64–70.

Pots, A. M., et al. (1999). Thermal aggregation of patatin studied in situ, *Journal of Agricultural and Food Chemistry, 47*(11), 4600–4605.

Qi, Y., et al. (2018). Mitigation effects of proanthocyanidins with different structures on acrylamide formation in chemical and fried potato crisp models. *Food Chemistry, 250*, 98–104.

Raigond, P., Jayanty, S. S., & Dutt, S. (2020). New health-promoting compounds in potatoes. In *Potato* (pp. 213–228). Springer.

Rogozińska, I., et al. (2005). The effect of different factors on the content of nitrate in some potato varieties, *Potato Research, 48*(3–4), 167–180.

Ruan, S., et al. (2021). Staple food and health: A comparative study of physiology and gut microbiota of mice fed with potato and traditional staple foods (corn, wheat and rice). *Foods & Function, 12*(3).

Ruark, M. D., Kelling, K. A., & Good, L. W. (2014). Environmental concerns of phosphorus management in potato production, *American Journal of Potato Research, 91*(2), 132–144.

Salvador, A. F., et al. (2019). Potato ingestion is as effective as carbohydrate gels to support prolonged cycling performance, *Journal of Applied Physiology, 127*(6), 1651–1659.

Sanders, L., et al. (2021). Effects of potato resistant starch intake on insulin sensitivity, related metabolic markers and appetite ratings in men and women at risk for type 2 diabetes: A pilot crossover randomised controlled trial, *Journal of Human Nutrition and Dietetics, 34*(1), 94–105.

Schwingshackl, L., et al. (2019). Potatoes and risk of chronic disease: A systematic review and dose-response meta-analysis. *European Journal of Nutrition, 58*(6), 2243–2251.

Shakya, R., & Navarre, D. A. (2008). LC-MS analysis of solanidane glycoalkaloid diversity among tubers of four wild potato species and three cultivars (Solanum tuberosum), *Journal of Agricultural and Food Chemistry, 56*(16), 6949–6958.

So, J., et al. (2020). Potato consumption and risk of cardio-metabolic diseases: Evidence mapping of observational studies, *Systematic Reviews, 9*(1), 1–9.

Sordini, B., et al. (2019). A quanti-qualitative study of a phenolic extract as a natural antioxidant in the frying processes. *Food Chemistry, 279*, 426–434.

Spooner, D. M., et al. (2005). A single domestication for potato based on multilocus amplified fragment length polymorphism genotyping. *Proceedings of the National Academy of Sciences of the United States of America, 102*(41), 14694.

Stushnoff, C., et al. (2008). Antioxidant properties of cultivars and selections from the Colorado potato breeding program. *American Journal of Potato Research, 85*(4), 267–276.

Sun, Y., Jiang, L., & Wei, D. (2013). Partial characterization, in vitro antioxidant and antiproliferative activities of patatin purified from potato fruit juice. *Food & Function, 4*(10), 1502–1511.

Thompson, M. D., et al. (2009). Functional food characteristics of potato cultivars (Solanum tuberosum L.): Phytochemical composition and inhibition of 1-methyl-1-nitrosourea induced breast cancer in rats, *Journal of Food Composition and Analysis, 22*(6), 571–576.

Tsang, C., et al. (2018). Antioxidant rich potato improves arterial stiffness in healthy adults, *Plant Foods for Human Nutrition, 73*(3), 203–208.

USDA and NASS. (2020). *Crop values 2019 summary*. 2020: USDA's National Agricultural Statistics Service.

Van Eck, J., et al. (2007). Enhancing beta-carotene content in potato by RNAi-mediated silencing of the beta-carotene hydroxylase gene, *American Journal of Potato Research, 84*(4), 331–342.

Vinson, J. A., et al. (2012). High-antioxidant potatoes: Acute in vivo antioxidant source and hypotensive agent in humans after supplementation to hypertensive subjects, *Journal of Agricultural and Food Chemistry, 60*(27), 6749–6754.

Waglay, A., & Karboune, S. (2016). Chapter 4 – Potato proteins: Functional food ingredients. In J. Singh & L. Kaur (Eds.), *Advances in potato chemistry and technology (second edition)* (pp. 75–104). Academic.

Wallace, T. C., Slavin, M., & Frankenfeld, C. L. (2016). Systematic review of anthocyanins and markers of cardiovascular disease, *Nutrients, 8*(1), 32.

Waltz, E. (2015). *USDA approves next-generation GM potato*. Nature Publishing.

Wang, L. L., & Xiong, Y. L. (2005). Inhibition of lipid oxidation in cooked beef patties by hydrolyzed potato protein is related to its reducing and radical scavenging ability. *Journal of Agricultural and Food Chemistry, 53*(23), 9186–9192.

Wang, Q., et al. (2016). Kukoamine A inhibits human glioblastoma cell growth and migration through apoptosis induction and epithelial-mesenchymal transition attenuation, *Scientific Reports, 6*(1), 1–13.

White, P. J., et al. (2017). Biofortifying Scottish potatoes with zinc, *Plant and Soil, 411*(1–2), 151–165.

Williams, J. S. E. (2005). Influence of variety and processing conditions on acrylamide levels in fried potato crisps. *Food Chemistry, 90*(4), 875–881.

Wu, J., et al. (2020). Prediction and identification of antioxidant peptides in potato protein hydrolysate. *Journal of Food Quality, 2020*, 8889555.

Yusuph, M., et al. (2003). Composition and properties of starches extracted from tubers of different potato varieties grown under the same environmental conditions, *Food Chemistry, 82*(2), 283–289.

Zhang, Y., et al. (2018). Potatoes consumption and risk of type 2 diabetes: A meta-analysis. *Iranian Journal of Public Health, 47*(11), 1627–1635.

Zhao, X., Andersson, M., & Andersson, R. (2018). Resistant starch and other dietary fiber components in tubers from a high-amylose potato, *Food Chemistry, 251*, 58–63.

Zhao, Q., et al. (2020). Kukoamine B ameliorate insulin resistance, oxidative stress, inflammation and other metabolic abnormalities in high-fat/high-fructose-fed rats, *Diabetes, Metabolic Syndrome and Obesity: Targets and Therapy, 13*, 1843.

Zhu, F., et al. (2010). Compositions of phenolic compounds, amino acids and reducing sugars in commercial potato varieties and their effects on acrylamide formation. *Journal of the Science of Food and Agriculture, 90*(13), 2254–2262.

Zhu, Y., Lasrado, J. A., & Hu, J. (2017). Potato protease inhibitor II suppresses postprandial appetite in healthy women: A randomized double-blind placebo-controlled trial. *Food & Function, 8*(5), 1988–1993.

Chapter 14
Grapes & Wine

Charlene Van Buiten

14.1 Introduction

Wine, a fermented, alcoholic beverage created from grapes, has retained global popularity since its ancient origins. It has been reported to serve a variety functions over the course of history, playing a role in social, religious and medicinal rituals, many of which are preserved in some form in the modern age. Wines, particularly those made from red grapes, are rich in bioactive compounds that have been associated with a variety of health benefits. As a "whole food", the consumption of red wine has been identified as one of the key components of the French Paradox, wherein the increased risk for coronary heart disease associated with a diet rich in saturated fats is offset by moderate intake of wine (Renaud & Lorgeril, 1992).

14.2 Cultural History

In the present day, wine can be found in many varieties and forms. Broadly, classifications of wine include table wines, such as traditional reds, whites or rosés, sparkling wines including Champagne, cava and spumante, and fortified wines like port, sherry and madeira, which require additional processing steps like aging and the addition of a distilled spirit to increase alcohol content. The majority of wines produced globally are made from carefully cultivated *Vitis vinifera* subsp. *vinifera* grapes, colloquially referred to as "wine grapes" (Jackson, 2016).

While the earliest record of grape and wine production dates back to 7000 B.C., viticulture and viniculture recognizable to present-day practices appear to have

C. Van Buiten (✉)
Colorado State University, Fort Collins, CO, USA
e-mail: Charlene.vanbuiten@colostate.edu

© The Author(s), under exclusive license to Springer Nature Switzerland AG 2022
J. P. Miller, C. Van Buiten (eds.), *Superfoods*, Food and Health,
https://doi.org/10.1007/978-3-030-93240-4_14

developed as grapevine cultivation spread westward from the Near East via Phoenician trading routes (Terral et al., 2010). Wine emerged as a documented staple in human culture with the ancient Greeks who, in their worship of Dionysus, the god of wine, would hold festivals celebrating the maturation of the wine made from the previous year's harvest (Robertson, 1993). The spread of the Roman empire across present-day Europe introduced *V. vinifera* and winemaking to Italy, Spain, Portugal and France, all of which have longstanding traditions of winemaking today (Terral et al., 2010) (Fig. 14.1).

Wine was adopted into religious rituals in the Middle Ages with the rise of Christianity, a symbolic tribute which is still used in many faiths today. This time period also saw remarkable growth in the intake of wine on a regular basis alongside or in the place of food. It has been suggested that the high acid and ethanol content of wine likely made the consumption of wine safer than the consumption of water. However, the quality of wine at this time was thought to be very poor due to improper sanitation and poor seals on storage vessels (Younger, 1966), leading to oxidation and secondary fermentations. Advances in wine production and quality can be attributed to its place in religious lore; monasteries were often tasked with providing wine for religious ceremonies but produced secular wine as well. Their strategies for viticulture and wine production developed over generations and spread with the establishment of new abbeys across Europe. The Cistercian abbeys of Burgundy and Bordeaux were regarded as a producers of high-quality wines and are credited with establishing the first wine cellars for long-term storage. As the Cistercians

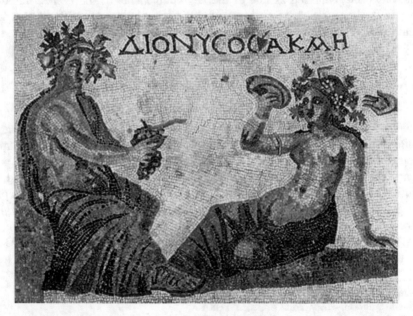

Fig. 14.1 Wine played a significant role in the culture of many civilizations, including ancient Greece. Festivals and artwork, such as this mosaic, featured Dionysus (left) or other mythological beings consuming grapes and wine

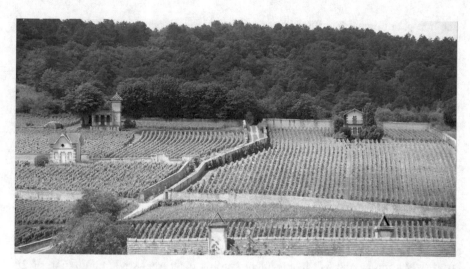

Fig. 14.2 The Burgundy region of France has long been associated with production and storage of fine wines. Vineyards established here in the Middle Ages still thrive today

spread across Europe, so did their traditions for winemaking (Estreicher, 2007) (Fig. 14.2).

Today, the wine industry is worth an estimated $326 billion U.S. globally, with an annual production volume of approximately 270 hectoliters (OIV, 2019) and the average American consuming 2.95 gallons per person per year (Wine Institute, 2019). The factors that drive consumption of wine in present time appear to be both physical and psychological; drinking wine has been reported to be socially motivated and most often associated with positive, pleasant feelings (Ferrarini et al., 2010; Taylor et al., 2018), and in a 2011 survey, 52% of wine drinkers reported that they believed wine was good for their health (St. James & Christodoulidou, 2011).

14.3 Wine: Current State of Research and Health Claims

Wine has a long history of use for medicinal purposes dating back to the writings of Hippocrates (460–370 B.C.E.), where it was prescribed as a diuretic, laxative, and general treatment against fatigue and stress (Jouanna & Allies, 2012), as well as an anesthetic and antiseptic agent as documented by Dioscorides (80 A.D.) and Galen (131–201 A.D.). In contrast to the perceived benefits of wine consumption, these early physicians also noted the negative effects of wine due to its alcohol content including both intoxication and hangovers.

In modern times, the investigation of the health benefits of wine focus on moderation when examined as a whole food, or cut out the alcoholic component of the beverage altogether, instead focusing on isolated phytochemicals found naturally in wine and grapes, known as polyphenols. Common polyphenols found in wine include phenolic acids, stilbenes, anthocyanins, which contribute to red and purple hues of red wines, and procyanidins, which contribute to the oral tactile sensation of astringency. These compounds are found naturally in the skin and seeds of grapes, and are extracted from crushed grapes over the course of fermentation (Kennedy & Peyrot, 2003). The antioxidant capabilities of these compounds have pushed them to the forefront of functional food research as potential mediators of inflammation and oxidative stress (Biasi et al., 2014; Georgiev et al., 2014; Giovinazzo & Grieco, 2015; Snopek et al., 2018).

14.3.1   Alcohol Consumption: Risk Vs. Benefit

It must be noted that alcohol in any form can have a negative impact on health. The Global Burden of Diseases, Injuries and Risk Factors Study, which collated data from 694 sources and 592 independent studies for a total study population of 28 million individuals, concluded that alcohol use was the seventh leading risk factor for death and disability in 2016, and the leading risk factor globally for individuals aged 15–49 years old (i.e., premature death). This statistic warns against even moderate alcohol consumption; there was no amount of alcohol consumption that was found to minimize health loss (Griswold et al., 2018). As a result, the consideration of wine as a whole food beneficial to health should be done with caution.

14.3.2   Cardiovascular Disease & "The French Paradox"

Wine is perhaps best known for its possible link to cardiovascular health via a phenomenon called "The French Paradox", wherein epidemiological studies have revealed an inverse relationship between incidence of coronary heart disease (CHD) and wine consumption (Leger et al., 1979), with France presenting the lowest CHD mortality rates despite an average diet notably high in saturated fats (Renaud & Lorgeril, 1992). The protective effects of red wine against cardiovascular disease have been attributed to its ability to reduce oxidative stress (Corredor et al., 2016; Copetti et al., 2018), preserve vascular (blood vessel) function (Siasos et al., 2014; da Luz et al., 2018), and reduce post-meal cholesterol oxidation (Natella et al., 2011).

In comparison to beer and spirits, moderate wine intake increased high density lipoprotein cholesterol (HDL) in individuals at risk for cardiovascular disease (Shai et al., 2004), suggesting that polyphenols are the bioactive component of wine in this context. However, a separate study where red wine was compared to drinking water with an equivalent dose of wine polyphenol extract (560 mg and 840 mg for female and male subjects, respectively) showed that alcohol does play a role in the cardioprotective effects associated with wine consumption (Hansen et al., 2005). The differential and possibly synergistic effects of red wine polyphenols and ethanol have been explored, with alcoholic red wines being shown to generally increase anti-inflammatory cytokines in high-risk individuals while dealcoholized red wine decreased proinflammatory cytokines (Chiva-Blanch et al., 2012).

Grape polyphenols, when consumed outside the context of wine as dietary supplements, have been shown to mitigate risk factors of cardiovascular disease including hypertension and atherosclerosis. Grapeseed extract consumed at rates of 150 and 300 mg per day over the course of 2 weeks reduced systolic and diastolic blood pressure in pre-hypertensive individuals (Clifton, 2004; Sivaprakasapillai et al., 2009), though no effect of grapeseed extract on blood pressure has been observed in healthy individuals (Sano et al., 2007). The anti-atherosclerotic properties of grape polyphenols include mediation of blood lipids and prevention of low-density lipoprotein (LDL) cholesterol oxidation. Grape juice has been shown to decrease total cholesterol and LDL while increasing high-density lipoprotein (HDL) in both healthy and hypercholesteremic individuals (Vinson et al., 2001; Castilla et al., 2006, 2008). The oxidation of LDL is also prevented by grape polyphenols; clinical trials where hemodialysis patients consumed 100 mL grape juice for 14 days showed 35–65% less oxidized LDL at the end of the study (Castilla et al., 2006, 2008).

14.3.3 Metabolic Syndrome & Type 2 Diabetes

Metabolic syndrome (MetS) is a cluster of symptoms including hypertension, hyperglycemia, dyslipidemia and obesity which increase an individual's risk for cardiovascular disease and type 2 diabetes. MetS affects approximately 1.4 billion people worldwide with increasing prevalence (O'Neill & O'Driscoll, 2015). The consumption of wine as a whole food has been studied for its effects on the development of MetS with both positive and negative outcomes.

In a cross-sectional study of 5801 elderly volunteers with high risk for cardiovascular disease, moderate red wine consumption (≥1 drink per day) was associated with lower risk of prevalent MetS and all MetS risk factors including abnormal waist circumference, low HDL cholesterol, hypertension and hyperglycemia. Interestingly, this association was stronger in women and former or current smokers (Tresserra-Rimbau et al., 2015). However, similar studies have failed to identify protective effects of wine consumption against MetS and instead establish a link with lifestyle factors such as education level, employment, civil status, physical activity, dietary intake and wellbeing (Rosell et al., 2003).

Type 2 diabetes (T2D) is a chronic metabolic disorder characterized by insulin resistance and impaired insulin secretion. Several epidemiological studies have shown that moderate wine consumption has a protective effect against the development of T2D, with "moderate" typically defined as 300 mL or two glasses of wine (Robertson, 2014). In each study, wine was associated with decreased risk of developing T2D overall (Stampfer et al., 1988; Hodge et al., 2006; Beulens et al., 2012; Cullmann et al., 2012; Rasouli et al., 2013) and was shown to be more protective against T2D development than other alcoholic beverages studied (Hodge et al., 2006; Beulens et al., 2012; Rasouli et al., 2013). However, these findings appear to also be dependent on other factors such as sex, lifestyle and predisposition to T2D (Conigrave et al., 2001).

One underlying mechanism identified for the protective effects of wine against T2D is the antioxidant activity of wine phenolics, which may reduce oxidative stress and inflammation. The intake of one serving of wine with a meal was shown to counteract the oxidative stress induced by eating (Ceriello et al., 1999). The long-term consumption of wine has been shown to be beneficial as well- moderate daily wine intake for one year reduced inflammatory markers associated with cardiac dysfunction (Marfella et al., 2006) and reduced insulin resistance (Gin et al., 1999; Napoli et al., 2005) in diabetic subjects.

Protection against MetS and T2D is better defined when examining the influence of grape phenolics not as a fraction of wine, but rather, when consumed as a dietary supplement. Supplementation with grape polyphenols has been shown to reverse MetS-associated inflammation in mice as well as prevent weight gain on a high-fat diet (Roopchand et al., 2015). These changes may be due to modification of the gut microbiome (Roopchand et al., 2015; Overall et al., 2017; Nash et al., 2018; Zhang et al., 2018), as well as direct radical scavenging in the gastrointestinal tract (Kuhn et al., 2018), a mechanism which has been shown to reverse MetS-associated hyperglycemia and production of reactive oxygen species (ROS) in a murine model of obesity (Van Buiten et al., 2021).

14.3.4   Chronic Respiratory Illness

Moderate intake of wine has been shown to protect against fatal respiratory diseases such as chronic obstructive pulmonary disease (COPD) (Kamholz, 2006). In two separate cohort studies relying on dietary recall to track wine consumption, the intake of the wine phenolic resveratrol from both white and red wine was positively associated with increased lung function (Siedlinski et al., 2012). Resveratrol's antioxidant and anti-inflammatory effects in respiratory illness have been explored in clinical and pre-clinical trials. Resveratrol targets key mediators of inflammation (Barnes, 2014; Bitterman & Chung, 2015) (Liu et al., 2014). Its efficacy has been demonstrated *in vitro* with cellular models of cigarette smoke-induced oxidative stress and *in vivo* using mouse models of COPD (Chen et al., 2016), but these benefits have not been corroborated in studies using human subjects.

When examined from the perspective of whole foods contributing resveratrol to the diet, a positive association was observed between the consumption of white wine and pulmonary function, but this association was not observed with red wine, which contains greater amounts of resveratrol per serving (Siedlinski et al., 2012). This suggests the possibility of confounding variables in the study, likely related to other lifestyle and dietary factors that were not controlled for in the analyses. As such, clear conclusions about the protective effects of wine against respiratory illnesses such as COPD cannot be drawn at this time.

14.3.5   Cancer

While cancer risk increases with alcohol intake, grape bioactives are thought to possess anti-carcinogenic effects and have been explored with respect to improving
human health in the form of dietary supplements. The efficacy of these compounds
in preventing or treating cancers vary based on type of cancer and disease model,
though it has been shown that regular flavonol intake is associated with decreased
cancer risk overall (Soobrattee et al., 2006). Specifically, breast cancer and colon
cancer risks are inversely associated with dietary intake of grape bioactives (Zhou
& Raffoul, 2012). The prevailing hypotheses for chemoprotection of grape polyphenols are related to their antioxidant activities and mediation of ROS (Sato et al.,
1999; Zhao et al., 1999). The anti-inflammatory capabilities of grape polyphenols
have also been studied; anti-tumor activity of grape polyphenols has been attributed
to their enhancement of lymphocyte proliferation and the upregulation of anti-
inflammatory cytokines including IL-2 and IFN-γ (Zhang et al., 2005).

The mechanistic data regarding anticarcinogenic effects of grape-derived compounds are based largely on *in vitro* studies, though their efficacy has been delin-
eated in some *in vivo* studies as well. Grapeseed proanthocyanidin supplementation
reduced lung tumors in predisposed mice and rats (Velmurugan et al., 2010; Sharma
et al., 2010). Targeted human studies in this area, however, are limited and inconsistent. While no benefit of grape products was observed in breast cancer patients
consuming grape seed proanthocyanidins, some specific modifications of molecular
pathways implicated in cancer have been demonstrated in human trials, including
reduced generation of ROS and reduced DNA damage upon daily consumption
wine polyphenols (57.2 mg/kg/day) (Giovannelli et al., 2000). Further studies are
required to understand the precise effects and mechanisms of grape polyphenols in
protection against various cancers.

14.4   Science Topics for Enhanced Understanding

14.4.1   Basic Grape Botany

Grapes are the berries of the flowering plant genus *Vitis*. They grow in clusters off
of deciduous, woody vines and, despite being classified as "red" or "white", can
grow in a variety of colors including black, crimson, green, blue and orange. The
color, shape and size of a given grape depends on its specific cultivar, growing conditions, and state of ripeness.

Like most fruits, grapes are made up mostly of water- about 74% in a ripe berry-
followed by 24% carbohydrates. Despite a relatively low contribution to the overall
composition of the grape, the compounds found in the remaining 2% of the grape
have a profound impact on the final product. These compounds include glycerol,

acids, phenolics, lipids, nitrogenous compounds and aroma compounds (Boulton et al., 1999).

Structurally, grapes have three primary features that influence wine production-the pulp, skin and seeds. By fresh weight, the pulp makes up the majority of the berry, at about 88% when ripe. Grape pulp is primarily water, but also includes simple, fermentable sugars, organic acids including tartaric and malic acid, and some flavor compounds. Notably, grape pulp is colorless. Pigmented wines, like reds and rosés, get their color from natural pigments known as anthocyanins, which are found in grape skins (Boulton et al., 1999) (Fig. 14.3).

Grape skins, which make up the outer layer of the berry, contribute pigmentation and flavor and aroma compounds to wines. White grapes are rich in phenolic acids which, while colorless, can oxidize to form brown pigments, whereas red grape skins primarily contribute anthocyanins, which can range from blue/purple to red/pink depending on the pH of the wine. When a wine is produced by allowing the juice from the pulp to remain in contact with the grape skins and seeds, anthocyanins become extracted from grape skins over the course of fermentation due to the increasing alcohol content of the solution. This change in alcohol content also

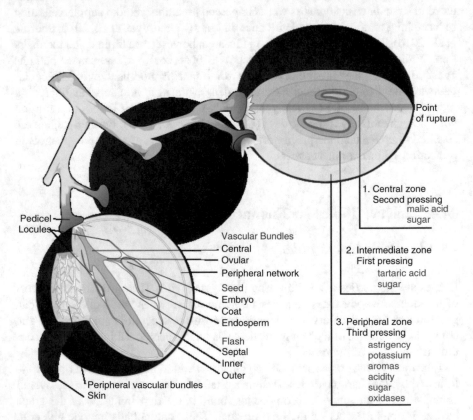

Fig. 14.3 A diagram of a wine grape. Pressing zones refer to areas of the grape which contribute different chemical compounds to juice upon pressing during the winemaking process

favors the extraction of colorless polyphenols known as procyanidins, which contribute to the astringent mouthfeel of red wines. In addition to being extracted from grape skin, procyanidins are also found in and extracted from grape seeds that are allowed to remain in contact with the juice during fermentation (Waterhouse, 2002).

14.4.2 Wine Polyphenol Chemistry

The previously discussed phenolic compounds found in grapes are often thought of as the prevailing bioactive component of wine due to their potent antioxidant capacity. However, these compounds also contribute to the overall quality of wines including the appearance, bitterness as astringency of the final product. Broadly, wine phenolics can be divided into two classifications- non-flavonoids and flavonoids. Each are found in both red and white wines, but in differing proportions. Overall, red wines contain greater concentrations of polyphenols in comparison to white wines with about 200 mg per glass of red wine versus 40 mg per glass of white wine (Boulton et al., 1999).

The non-flavonoids found in wine include stilbenes, hydroxycinnamic acids, hydrolyzable tannins and benzoic acids. Stilbenes, found in the skins of grapes, include the bioactive compound resveratrol, which has been associated with many of the previously discussed health benefits of wine. Resveratrol is found in both red and white grapes, though the concentration in red grapes is often significantly higher, at 7 mg/L and 0.5 mg/L, respectively (Romero-Pérez et al., 1996). Hydroxycinnamic acids are small phenolic molecules found in both red and white grapes that play a significant role in the discoloration of white wines, as the oxidation of hydroxycinnamic acids, such as caffeic acid, results in the formation of compounds known as quinones, which cause browning (Cheynier et al., 1990). Hydrolyzable tannins and benzoic acids, uniquely, affect the flavor and mouthfeel of wine but are not derived from grapes, rather, they are extracted from wood over the course of barrel aging. Hydrolyzable tannins are large, branched molecules that can be hydrolyzed into their monomeric subunits of benzoic acids, which are relatively stable in wines over time (Quinn & Singleton, 1985).

Wine flavonoids include flavonols, anthocyanins and flavanols. Flavonols exist in three simple forms in grapes- quercetin, myricetin and kaempferol; however, diversity of these compounds arises through interactions with sugars and the formation of glycosides (Waterhouse, 2002). These compounds are of particular importance to grapes during the growth and ripening process, as they protect the berry from potentially harmful UV light (Price et al., 1995). Anthocyanins are flavonoids which contribute color to red wine. Found in the skins of grapes, anthocyanins comprise an anthocyanidin stabilized through glycoside formation (Waterhouse, 2002). Common anthocyanins found in red wine are the glycosidic forms of malvidin, cyanidin, peonidin, petunidin and delphinidin. The precise hue of wine imparted by these compounds is dependent on concentration of anthocyanins, proportions of individual compounds and pH. Higher pH wines tend to be more violet in color, whereas lower pH wines favor crimson red hues (Boulton et al., 1999). The final category of flavonoids found in wine, known as flavanols or flavan-3-ols, largely contribute to astringency and mouthfeel of the wine. Monomeric flavan-3-ols found in wine are known as catechins and exist in various forms based on substitution of their phenolic rings with gallate groups. These monomers can condense to form oligomeric and polymeric compounds known as proanthocyanidins and condensed tannins, respectively. These compounds typically make up the greatest proportion of phenolics found in wines, and the proportion increases over the course of aging as the molecules continue to condense (Waterhouse, 2002). Proanthocyanidins and condensed tannins impart astringency in wine via interaction with salivary proteins. This interaction results in the formation of protein-polyphenol complexes and subsequent protein precipitation. Astringency in a wine can be "softened" through the addition of fining agents such as gelatin, casein and polyvinylpolypyrrolidone prior to bottling or sale. These fining agents pre-emptively remove a portion of the proanthocyanidins and tannins from solution, making them less abundant and available for interaction with salivary proteins upon consumption (Ribereau-Gayon et al., 2006) (Fig. 14.4).

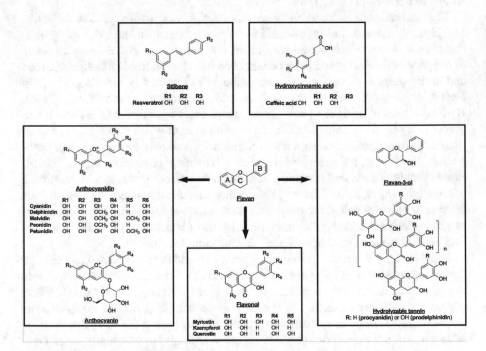

Fig. 14.4 Common phenolic compounds found in wine. The composition and concentrations of each depend on parameters such as grape varietal, processing conditions and storage conditions. These compounds contribute to the overall quality of the wine, affecting characteristics such as color, mouthfeel and health benefits

14.5 Current Issues

Mirroring most food trends over the last several decades, the wine industry has undergone a shift towards sustainable practices and the production of wines labeled as "natural", "organic" and "biodynamic" (Yiridoe et al., 2005; Döring et al., 2019). Sustainability concerns in viticulture and enology stem from environmental factors as well as economic ones- while climate change, water availability and energy use threaten the industry (Flores, 2018), consumer demand demonstrates the potential for greater profit margins on products produced with specialty labeling guaranteeing a greater degree of environmental-friendliness and production transparency (Mann et al., 2012; Amato et al., 2017; Schäufele & Hamm, 2017) (Fig. 14.5).

Per the International Organization of Vine and Wine, sustainable viticulture is defined as a "global strategy on the scale of the grape production and processing systems, incorporating at the same time the economic sustainability of structures and territories, producing quality products, considering requirements of precision in sustainable viticulture, risks to the environment, product safety and consumer health and valuing of heritage, historical, cultural, ecological and aesthetic aspects" (OIV, 2004). Guidelines have been set in place for sustainable production, processing and packaging of wines (OIV, 2008).

Organic practices in winemaking vary based on the country the wine was produced in; for example, the United States differentiates between "organic wine" versus "wine made with organic grapes" based on the percentage of organic grapes in the product and the application of sulfur dioxide for preservation purposes (Cravero, 2019). The labeling of these wines also requires inspection by the United States Department of Agriculture. Biodynamic practices on the other hand, are not regulated at the federal level and reflect a more holistic approach to agriculture than

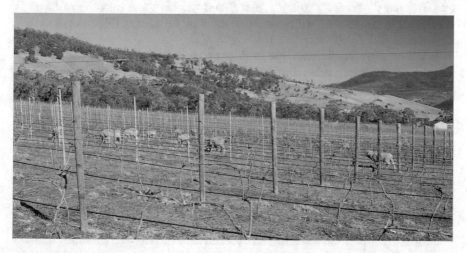

Fig. 14.5 Biodynamic viticulture includes sustainable strategies for crop management. At Stefano Lubiana Wines/Granton Vineyard in Tasmania, Australia, sheep graze in the vineyard as a sustainable and organic strategy for weed control

organic practices, which focus primarily on the elimination of synthetic processing agents (Castellini et al., 2017). Broadly, the three principles of biodynamic are maintenance of soil fertility, the growth of healthy, pest- and disease-resistant plants, and the production of high-quality food products. These principles are attained through the employment of cultivation strategies like cover crops and natural fertilizers at the vineyard level, and the elimination of many popular processing ingredients and additives during vinification including certain yeasts, enzymes, bacteria and fining agents (Cravero, 2019).

14.6 Wine and Food

Though wine can be used as an ingredient in some prepared meals, it is most often presented alongside foods to enhance a dish by providing either complementary or congruent features. The science of wine pairing is based on the interplay between sensorial aspects of both the food and the wine. These sensorial aspects are classified into three categories- components, texture and flavors.

The "components" of a food or wine relate to basic, primary characteristics including acidity, sweetness and effervescence in a wine and sweetness, saltiness, bitterness and sourness in a food. The term "texture" refers to the mouthfeel, or oral tactile sensation of the item in question. For wines, the astringency conferred by tannins, softness of oak aging, burn of alcohol and "body" contributed by glycerol content all make up the overall texture. In a food, texture is defined by the fattiness, cooking method or body of the meal. Finally, "flavor" refers to specific characteristics of aroma and taste resulting from retronasal processes during consumption. Wine flavors are typically based on a specific lexicon, including common descriptors like "oaky", "fruity", "spicy", "nutty" and "herbal", and intensity of flavor is considered in conjunction with specific descriptors for pairing (Noble et al., 1987; Kustos et al., 2020).

While creating unique favorable pairings can be a complex process specific to a given food or wine, some traditional recommendations prevail including the following:

- Avoid pairing red wine with seafood/white fish (Simon, 1996), as iron chelation can cause the formation of fishy and metallic off-aromas (Tamura et al., 2009)
- Pair jammy red wines like Zinfandel with high moisture cheeses for a dessert-like perception (Spence, 2020)
- Wine with buttery aromas can be enhanced by cheeses with similarly buttery flavors (Madrigal-Galan & Heymann, 2006)
- Astringent, high-tannin red wines can reduce the perception of fattiness in a meal (des Gachons et al., 2012)
- Acidic, mineral white wines like an unoaked Chablis pair well with salty seafood dishes, like oysters (Lorman 2020)

References

Amato, M., Ballco, P., López-Galán, B., et al. (2017). Exploring consumers' perception and willingness to pay for "non-added sulphite" wines through experimental auctions: A case study in Italy and Spain. *Wine Economics and Policy, 6*, 146–154. https://doi.org/10.1016/j.wep.2017.10.002

Barnes, P. J. (2014). Cellular and molecular mechanisms of chronic obstructive pulmonary disease. *Clinics in Chest Medicine, 35*, 71–86. https://doi.org/10.1016/j.ccm.2013.10.004

Beulens, J. W. J., Van der Schouw, Y. T., Bergmann, M. M., et al. (2012). Alcohol consumption and risk of type 2 diabetes in European men and women: Influence of beverage type and body sizeThe EPIC-InterAct study. *Journal of Internal Medicine, 272*, 358–370. https://doi.org/10.1111/j.1365-2796.2012.02532.x

Biasi, F., Deiana, M., Guina, T., et al. (2014). Wine consumption and intestinal redox homeostasis. *Redox Biology, 2*, 795–802. https://doi.org/10.1016/j.redox.2014.06.008

Bitterman, J. L., & Chung, J. H. (2015). Metabolic effects of resveratrol: Addressing the controversies. *Cellular and Molecular Life Sciences, 72*, 1473–1488. https://doi.org/10.1007/s00018-014-1808-8

Boulton, R. B., Singleton, V. L., Bisson, L. F., & Kunkee, R. E. (1999). *Principles and practices of winemaking*. Springer.

Castellini, A., Mauracher, C., & Troiano, S. (2017). An overview of the biodynamic wine sector. *Int J Wine Res, 9*, 1–11. https://doi.org/10.2147/IJWR.S69126

Castilla, P., Echarri, R., Dávalos, A., et al. (2006). Concentrated red grape juice exerts antioxidant, hypolipidemic, and antiinflammatory effects in both hemodialysis patients and healthy subjects. *The American Journal of Clinical Nutrition, 84*, 252–262. https://doi.org/10.1093/ajcn/84.1.252

Castilla, P., Dávalos, A., Teruel, J. L., et al. (2008). Comparative effects of dietary supplementation with red grape juice and vitamin E on production of superoxide by circulating neutrophil NADPH oxidase in hemodialysis patients. *The American Journal of Clinical Nutrition, 87*, 1053–1061. https://doi.org/10.1093/ajcn/87.4.1053

Ceriello, A., Bortolotti, N., Motz, E., et al. (1999). Meal-generated oxidative stress in diabetes. The protective effect of red wine. *Diabetes Care, 22*, 2084–2085.

Chen, J., Yang, X., Zhang, W., et al. (2016). Therapeutic effects of resveratrol in a mouse model of LPS and cigarette smoke-induced COPD. *Inflammation, 39*, 1949–1959. https://doi.org/10.1007/s10753-016-0430-3

Cheynier, V., Rigaud, J., Souquet, J.-M., et al. (1990). Must browning in relation to the behavior of phenolic compounds during oxidation. *American Journal of Enology and Viticulture, 41*, 346.

Chiva-Blanch, G., Urpi-Sarda, M., Llorach, R., et al. (2012). Differential effects of polyphenols and alcohol of red wine on the expression of adhesion molecules and inflammatory cytokines related to atherosclerosis: A randomized clinical trial. *The American Journal of Clinical Nutrition, 95*, 326–334. https://doi.org/10.3945/ajcn.111.022889

Clifton, P. M. (2004). Effect of grape seed extract and quercetin on cardiovascular and endothelial parameters in high-risk subjects. *Journal of Biomedicine & Biotechnology, 2004*, 272–278. https://doi.org/10.1155/S1110724304403088

Conigrave, K. M., Hu, B. F., Camargo, C. A., et al. (2001). A prospective study of drinking patterns in relation to risk of type 2 diabetes among men. *Diabetes, 50*, 2390–2395. https://doi.org/10.2337/diabetes.50.10.2390

Copetti, C., Franco, F. W., Machado, E. D. R., et al. (2018). Acute consumption of Bordo grape juice and wine improves serum antioxidant status in healthy individuals and inhibits reactive oxygen species production in human neuron-like cells. *Journal of Nutrition and Metabolism, 2018*. https://doi.org/10.1155/2018/4384012

Corredor, Z., Rodríguez-Ribera, L., Coll, E., et al. (2016). Unfermented grape juice reduce genomic damage on patients undergoing hemodialysis. *Food and Chemical Toxicology, 92*, 1–7. https://doi.org/10.1016/j.fct.2016.03.016

Cravero, M. C. (2019). Organic and biodynamic wines quality and characteristics: A review. *Food Chemistry, 295*, 334–340. https://doi.org/10.1016/j.foodchem.2019.05.149

Cullmann, M., Hilding, A., & Östenson, C. G. (2012). Alcohol consumption and risk of pre-diabetes and type 2 diabetes development in a Swedish population. *Diabetic Medicine, 29*, 441–452. https://doi.org/10.1111/j.1464-5491.2011.03450.x

da Luz, P. L., Favarato, D., Moriguchi, E. H., et al. (2018). Red wine consumption, coronary calcification, and long-term clinical evolution. *Brazilian Journal of Medical and Biological Research, 51.*

des Gachons, C. P., Mura, E., Speziale, C., et al. (2012). Opponency of astringent and fat sensa-tions. *Current Biology, 22*, R829–R830. https://doi.org/10.1016/j.cub.2012.08.017

Döring, J., Collins, C., Frisch, M., & Kauer, R. (2019). Organic and biodynamic viticulture affect biodiversity and properties of vine and wine: A systematic quantitative review. *American Journal of Enology and Viticulture, 70*, 221–242. https://doi.org/10.5344/ajev.2019.18047

Estreicher, S. K. (2007). *Wine: From Neolithic times to the 21st century.* Algora Publishing.

Ferrarini, R., Carbognin, C., Casarotti, E. M., et al. (2010). The emotional response to wine consumption. *Food Quality and Preference, 21*, 720–725. https://doi.org/10.1016/j.foodqual.2010.06.004

Flores, S. S. (2018). What is sustainability in the wine world? A cross-country analysis of wine sustainability frameworks. *Journal of Cleaner Production, 172*, 2301–2312. https://doi.org/10.1016/j.jclepro.2017.11.181

Georgiev, V., Ananga, A., & Tsolova, V. (2014). Recent advances and uses of grape flavonoids as nutraceuticals. *Nutrients, 6*, 391–415. https://doi.org/10.3390/nu6010391

Gin, H., Rigalleau, V., Caubet, O., et al. (1999). Effects of red wine, tannic acid, or ethanol on glucose tolerance in non-insulin-dependent diabetic patients and on starch digestibility in vitro. *Metabolism, 48*, 1179–1183. https://doi.org/10.1016/S0026-0495(99)90135-X

Giovannelli, L., Testa, G., De Filippo, C., et al. (2000). Effect of complex polyphenols and tannins from red wine on DNA oxidative damage of rat colon mucosa in vivo. *European Journal of Nutrition, 39*, 207–212. https://doi.org/10.1007/s003940070013

Giovinazzo, G., & Grieco, F. (2015). Functional properties of grape and wine polyphenols. *Plant Foods for Human Nutrition, 70*, 454–462. https://doi.org/10.1007/s11130-015-0518-1

Griswold, M. G., Fullman, N., Hawley, C., et al. (2018). Alcohol use and burden for 195 countries and territories, 1990-2016: A systematic analysis for the global burden of disease study 2016. *Lancet, 392*, 1015–1035. https://doi.org/10.1016/S0140-6736(18)31310-2

Hansen, A. S., Marckmann, P., Dragsted, L. O., et al. (2005). Effect of red wine and red grape extract on blood lipids, haemostatic factors, and other risk factors for cardiovascular disease. *European Journal of Clinical Nutrition, 59*, 449–455. https://doi.org/10.1038/sj.ejcn.1602107

Hodge, A. M., English, D. R., O'Dea, K., & Giles, G. G. (2006). Alcohol intake, consumption pat-tern and beverage type, and the risk of type 2 diabetes. *Diabetic Medicine, 23*, 690–697. https://doi.org/10.1111/j.1464-5491.2006.01864.x

Jackson, R. (2016). Viticulture. In *Reference module in food science.* Elsevier.

Jouanna, J., & Allies, N. (2012). Wine and medicine in ancient Greece. In P. van der Eijk (Ed.), *Greek medicine from Hippocrates to Galen* (pp. 173–194). Brill.

Kamholz, S. L. (2006). Wine, spirits and the lung: Good, bad or indifferent? *Transactions of the American Clinical and Climatological Association, 117*, 129–145.

Kennedy, B. Y. J. A., & Peyrot, C. (2003). Phenolic extraction in red wine production. *Winemaking*, pp 1–5.

Kuhn, P., Kalariya, H. M., Poulev, A., et al. (2018). Grape polyphenols reduce gut-localized reac-tive oxygen species associated with the development of metabolic syndrome in mice. *PLoS One, 13.* https://doi.org/10.1371/journal.pone.0198716

Kustos, M., Heymann, H., Jeffery, D. W., et al. (2020). Intertwined: What makes food and wine pairings appropriate? *Food Research International, 136*, 109463. https://doi.org/10.1016/j.foodres.2020.109463

Leger, A. S. S., Cochrane, A. L., & Moore, F. (1979). Factors associated with cardiac mortality in developed countries with particular reference to the consumption of wine. *Lancet, 313*, 1017–1020. https://doi.org/10.1016/S0140-6736(79)92765-X

Liu, H., Ren, J., Chen, H., et al. (2014). Resveratrol protects against cigarette smoke-induced oxidative damage and pulmonary inflammation. *Journal of Biochemical and Molecular Toxicology, 28*, 465–471. https://doi.org/10.1002/jbt.21586

Lorman, M. (2020). *What wine to drink with oysters*. DCanter. https://www.dcanterwines.com/blogs/wine-life/what-to-drink-with-oysters/. Accessed 30 Mar 2021.

Madrigal-Galan, B., & Heymann, H. (2006). Sensory effects of consuming cheese prior to evaluating red wine flavor. *American Journal of Enology and Viticulture, 57*, 12–22.

Mann, S., Ferjani, A., & Reissig, L. (2012). What matters to consumers of organic wine? *British Food Journal, 114*, 272–284. https://doi.org/10.1108/00070701211202430

Marfella, R., Cacciapuoti, F., Siniscalchi, M., et al. (2006). Effect of moderate red wine intake on cardiac prognosis after recent acute myocardial infarction of subjects with type 2 diabetes mellitus. *Diabetic Medicine, 23*, 974–981. https://doi.org/10.1111/j.1464-5491.2006.01886.x

Napoli, R., Cozzolino, D., Guardasole, V., et al. (2005). Red wine consumption improves insulin resistance but not endothelial function in type 2 diabetic patients. *Metabolism, 54*, 306–313. https://doi.org/10.1016/j.metabol.2004.09.010

Nash, V., Ranadheera, C. S., Georgousopoulou, E. N., et al. (2018). The effects of grape and red wine polyphenols on gut microbiota – A systematic review. *Food Research International, 113*, 277–287. https://doi.org/10.1016/j.foodres.2018.07.019

Natella, F., MacOne, A., Ramberti, A., et al. (2011). Red wine prevents the postprandial increase in plasma cholesterol oxidation products: A pilot study. *The British Journal of Nutrition, 105*, 1718–1723. https://doi.org/10.1017/S0007114510005544

Noble, A. C., Arnold, R. A., Buechsenstein, J., et al. (1987). Modification of a standardized system of wine aroma terminology. *American Journal of Enology and Viticulture, 38*, 143–146.

O'Neill, S., & O'Driscoll, L. (2015). Metabolic syndrome: A closer look at the growing epidemic and its associated pathologies. *Obesity Reviews, 16*, 1–12. https://doi.org/10.1111/obr.12229

OIV. (2004). *Resolution CST 1/2004 – Development of sustainable vitiviniculture*. Paris, France.

OIV. (2008). *Resolution CST 1/2008 – OIV guidelines for sustainable vitiviniculture: Production, processing and packaging of products*. Paris, France.

OIV. (2019). *2019 Statistical report on world vitiviniculture*.

Overall, J., Bonney, S. A., Wilson, M., et al. (2017). Metabolic effects of berries with structurally diverse anthocyanins. *International Journal of Molecular Sciences, 18*. https://doi.org/10.3390/ijms18020422

Price, S. F., Breen, P. J., Valladao, M., & Watson, B. T. (1995). Cluster sun exposure and quercetin in pinot noir grapes and wine. *American Journal of Enology and Viticulture, 46*, 187–194.

Quinn, M. K., & Singleton, V. L. (1985). Isolation and identification of Ellagitannins from white oak wood and an estimation of their roles in wine. *American Journal of Enology and Viticulture, 36*, 148–155.

Rasouli, B., Ahlbom, A., Andersson, T., et al. (2013). Alcohol consumption is associated with reduced risk of Type2 diabetes and autoimmune diabetes in adults: Results from the Nord-Trøndelag health study. *Diabetic Medicine, 30*, 56–64. https://doi.org/10.1111/j.1464-5491.2012.03713.x

Renaud, S., & De Lorgeril, M. (1992). Wine, alcohol, platelets and the French Paradox for coronary heart disease. *Lancet, 339*, 1523–1526.

Ribereau-Gayon, P., Glories, Y., Maujean, A., & Dubourdieu, D. (2006). *Handbook of Enology – The chemistry of wine stabilization and treatments* (2nd ed.). Wiley.

Robertson, N. (1993). Athens 'festival of the new wine festival Anthesteria is one of Athens' most renowned, coming, 95, 197–250.

Robertson, R. P. (2014). Red wine and diabetes health: Getting skin in the game. *Diabetes, 63*, 31–38. https://doi.org/10.2337/db13-1318

Romero-Pérez, A. I., Lamuela-Raventós, R. M., Waterhouse, A. L., & de la Torre-Boronat, M. C. (1996). Levels of cis- and trans-resveratrol and their glucosides in white and Rosé

Vitis vinifera wines from Spain. *Journal of Agricultural and Food Chemistry, 44*, 2124–2128. https://doi.org/10.1021/jf9507654

Roopchand, D. E., Carmody, R. N., Kuhn, P., et al. (2015). Dietary polyphenols promote growth of the gut bacterium akkermansia muciniphila and attenuate high-fat diet-induced metabolic syndrome. *Diabetes, 64*, 2847–2858. https://doi.org/10.2337/db14-1916

Rosell, M., de Faire, U., & Hellénius, M. L. (2003). Low prevalence of the metabolic syndrome in wine drinkers – Is it the alcohol beverage or the lifestyle? *European Journal of Clinical Nutrition, 57*, 227–234. https://doi.org/10.1038/sj.ejcn.1601548

Sano, A., Uchida, R., Saito, M., et al. (2007). Beneficial effects of grape seed extract on malondialdehyde-modified LDL. *Journal of Nutritional Science and Vitaminology (Tokyo), 53*, 174–182. https://doi.org/10.3177/jnsv.53.174

Sato, M., Maulik, G., Ray, P. S., et al. (1999). Cardioprotective effects of grape seed proantho-cyanidin against ischemic reperfusion injury. *Journal of Molecular and Cellular Cardiology, 31*(6), 1289–1297.

Schäufele, I., & Hamm, U. (2017). Consumers' perceptions, preferences and willingness-to-pay for wine with sustainability characteristics: A review. *Journal of Cleaner Production, 147*, 379–394. https://doi.org/10.1016/j.jclepro.2017.01.118

Shai, I., Rimm, E. B., Schulze, M. B., et al. (2004). Moderate alcohol intake and markers of inflammation and endothelial dysfunction among diabetic men. *Diabetologia, 47*, 1760–1767. https://doi.org/10.1007/s00125-004-1526-0

Sharma, S. D., Meeran, S. M., & Katiyar, S. K. (2010). Proanthocyanidins inhibit in vitro and in vivo growth of human non–small cell lung cancer cells by inhibiting the prostaglandin E(2) and prostaglandin E(2) receptors. *Molecular Cancer Therapeutics, 9*, 569–580. https://doi.org/10.1158/1535-7163.MCT-09-0638

Siasos, G., Tousoulis, D., Kokkou, E., et al. (2014). Favorable effects of concord grape juice on endothelial function and arterial stiffness in healthy smokers. *American Journal of Hypertension, 27*, 38–45. https://doi.org/10.1093/ajh/hpt176

Siedlinski, M., Boer, J. M. A., Smit, H. A., et al. (2012). Dietary factors and lung function in the general population: Wine and resveratrol intake. *The European Respiratory Journal, 39*, 385–391. https://doi.org/10.1183/09031936.00184110

Simon, J. (1996). Rules, & how to break them. In *Wine with food* (pp. 10–19). Octopus Publishing.

Sivaprakasapillai, B., Edirisinghe, I., Randolph, J., et al. (2009). Effect of grape seed extract on blood pressure in subjects with the metabolic syndrome. *Metabolism, 58*, 1743–1746. https://doi.org/10.1016/j.metabol.2009.05.030

Snopek, L., Mlcek, J., Sochorova, L., et al. (2018). Contribution of red wine consumption to human health protection. *Molecules, 23*, 1–16. https://doi.org/10.3390/molecules23071684

Soobrattee, M. A., Bahorun, T., & Aruoma, O. I. (2006). Chemopreventive actions of polyphenolic compounds in cancer. *BioFactors, 27*, 19–35. https://doi.org/10.1002/biof.5520270103

Spence, C. (2020). Food and beverage flavour pairing: A critical review of the literature. *Food Research International, 133*, 109124. https://doi.org/10.1016/j.foodres.2020.109124

St. James, M., & Christodoulidou, N. (2011). Factors influencing wine consumption in Southern California consumers. *International Journal of Wine Business Research, 23*, 36–48. https://doi.org/10.1108/17511061111121399

Stampfer, M. J., Colditz, G. A., Willett, W. C., et al. (1988). A prospective study of moderate alcohol drinking and risk of diabetes in women. *American Journal of Epidemiology, 128*, 549–558. https://doi.org/10.1093/oxfordjournals.aje.a115002

Tamura, T., Taniguchi, K., Suzuki, Y., et al. (2009). Iron is an essential cause of fishy aftertaste formation in wine and seafood pairing. *Journal of Agricultural and Food Chemistry, 57*, 8550–8556. https://doi.org/10.1021/jf901656k

Taylor, J. J., Bing, M., Reynolds, D., et al. (2018). Motivation and personal involvement leading to wine consumption. *International Journal of Contemporary Hospitality Management, 30*, 702–719. https://doi.org/10.1108/IJCHM-06-2016-0335

Terral, J. F., Tabard, E., Bouby, L., et al. (2010). Evolution and history of grapevine (Vitis vinifera) under domestication: New morphometric perspectives to understand seed domestication syndrome and reveal origins of ancient European cultivars. *Annals of Botany, 105*, 443–455. https://doi.org/10.1093/aob/mcp298

Tresserra-Rimbau, A., Medina-Remón, A., Lamuela-Raventós, R. M., et al. (2015). Moderate red wine consumption is associated with a lower prevalence of the metabolic syndrome in the PREDIMED population. *The British Journal of Nutrition, 113*, S121–S130. https://doi.org/10.1017/S0007114514003262

Van Buiten, C. B., Wu, G., Lam, Y. Y., et al. (2021). Elemental iron modifies the redox environment of the gastrointestinal tract: A novel therapeutic target and test for metabolic syndrome. *Free Radical Biology & Medicine, 168*, 203–213. https://doi.org/10.1016/j.freeradbiomed.2021.03.032

Velmurugan, B., Singh, R. P., Agarwal, R., & Agarwal, C. (2010). Dietary-feeding of grape seed extract prevents azoxymethane-induced colonic aberrant crypt foci formation in fischer 344 rats. *Molecular Carcinogenesis, 49*, 641–652. https://doi.org/10.1002/mc.20643

Vinson, J. A., Proch, J., & Bose, P. (2001). MegaNatural® gold grapeseed extract: In vitro antioxidant and in vivo human supplementation studies. *Journal of Medicinal Food, 4*, 17–26. https://doi.org/10.1089/10966200152053677

Waterhouse, A. L. (2002). Wine phenolics. *Annals of the New York Academy of Sciences, 957*, 21–36. https://doi.org/10.1080/09571269508718028

Wine Institute. (2019.) *US Wine Consumption*. San Francisco.

Yiridoe, E. K., Bonti-Ankomah, S., & Martin, R. C. (2005). Comparison of consumer perceptions and preference toward organic versus conventionally produced foods: A review and update of the literature. *Renewable Agriculture and Food Systems, 20*, 193–205. https://doi.org/10.1079/raf2005113

Younger, W. (1966). *Gods, men and wine, first*. World Publishing.

Zhang, X. Y., Li, W. G., Wu, Y. J., et al. (2005). Proanthocyanidin from grape seeds potentiates anti-tumor activity of doxorubicin via immunomodulatory mechanism. *International Immunopharmacology, 5*, 1247–1257. https://doi.org/10.1016/j.intimp.2005.03.004

Zhang, L., Carmody, R. N., Kalariya, H. M., et al. (2018). Grape proanthocyanidin-induced intestinal bloom of Akkermansia muciniphila is dependent on its baseline abundance and precedes activation of host genes related to metabolic health. *The Journal of Nutritional Biochemistry, 56*, 142–151. https://doi.org/10.1016/j.jnutbio.2018.02.009

Zhao, J., Wang, J., Chen, Y., & Agarwal, R. (1999). Anti-tumor-promoting activity of a polyphenolic fraction isolated from grape seeds in the mouse skin two-stage initiation-promotion protocol and identification of procyanidin B5-3′-gallate as the most effective antioxidant constituent. *Carcinogenesis, 20*, 1737–1745. https://doi.org/10.1093/carcin/20.9.1737

Zhou, K., & Raffoul, J. J. (2012). Potential anticancer properties of grape antioxidants. *Journal of Oncology, 2012*. https://doi.org/10.1155/2012/803294

Index